COWBOYS AND INDIAN

COWBOYS AND INDIAN
A Doctor's First Year in Texas

SANDIP V. MATHUR

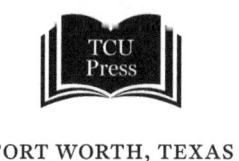

FORT WORTH, TEXAS

Library of Congress Cataloging-in-Publication Data

Names: Mathur, Sandip, 1961– author.
Title: Cowboys and Indian : a doctor's first year in Texas / Sandip Mathur.
Description: Fort Worth, Texas : [TCU Press], [2021]
Identifiers: LCCN 2021007090 (print) | LCCN 2021007091 (ebook) |
    ISBN 9780875657721 (paperback) | ISBN 9780875657820 (ebook)
Subjects: LCSH: Mathur, Sandip, 1961– | East Indian American physicians Texas—
    Biography. | Physicians—Texas—Biography. | East Indian Americans—Texas—
    Biography. | Immigrant families—Texas—Biography. | Rural health services—
    Texas, West. | Physician and patient—Texas, West. | LCGFT: Creative nonfiction.
    | Autobiographies.
Classification: LCC R154.M298765A3 2021 (print) |
    LCC R154.M298765A3 2021 (ebook) | DDC 610.92 [B]—dc23
LC record available at https://lccn.loc.gov/2021007090
LC ebook record available at https://lccn.loc.gov/2021007091

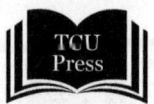

TCU Box 298300
Fort Worth, Texas 76129
To order books: 1.800.826.8911

On the cover: Photograph by Michelle Hanna.
Texas road map detail, Texas Department of Transportation.

To Maya, who made everything possible,
and
Santosh, Kamla, and the two Vijays.

CONTENTS

Prologue

I have always wanted to be a doctor, nothing but a doctor.

My parents are doctors. My grandfather, uncles, aunts, and cousins on both sides were surgeons, internists, obstetricians and gynecologists, pediatricians, and professors. I loved hearing about their lives: their patients, their struggles, their victories, and their defeats. Naturally, I was delighted and relieved when I was admitted to medical school in 1979. I was eighteen years old; that was the norm in India. Four years later, I emerged with my degree.

I decided to go to London, England, for training in internal medicine. With my father's connections, I was able to find a position in a London teaching hospital. I passed my certification exams in general internal medicine, and then specialized in liver disease.

In 1988, during a trip to India, I was introduced to Maya, a dazzling architect from my hometown. We were married later that year, and she joined me in London. Our older daughter, Priya, was born there in 1990.

I wanted to be a professor like my father. I wanted to look after patients, perform research, write papers, and teach medical students and young doctors. My training in liver diseases had been too specialized, so I decided to train in general gastroenterology, of which liver diseases is a part. But there was a problem: I could not find a suitable position in England. My father's colleague called her professor in Houston for advice. He told her that a fellowship training position in general gastroenterology had unexpectedly become available. I flew down for an interview, and they offered me the fellowship. I accepted immediately.

So Maya, Priya, and I moved to Houston in December 1990. I completed a fellowship in general gastroenterology in 1993.

Houston was very different from London. We adjusted easily; the people and the weather reminded us of India. The people were friendly, the climate warm and sunny, and there were many more academic opportunities than in England or India. So, at the end of the fellowship, I applied for a Texas medical license and hunted for research and teaching jobs.

I hit a wall. I was told that the training in London was not acceptable for licensure. I needed a medical license to get a job, and for that, I had to complete another residency program here in the United States. So, while the others in my fellowship program launched their careers as specialists, I went back for two years to complete a second round of training in basic internal medicine before finally obtaining my Texas medical license.

Then only one deficiency remained: we needed green cards.

A handful of federal agencies offered green cards to doctors. The Veterans Administration helped the VA hospitals, and the US Department of Agriculture helped rural communities. I was rejected by three academic VA hospitals, but, thanks to the USDA, a small, rural town in Texas was able to offer me a job and sponsorship for naturalization. I had four months left on my visa. I abandoned academics and plunged into practice in small-town Texas, desperate to succeed.

This is the account of my first year in medical practice. It was over twenty years ago. I want to share the excitement of medicine in the rural world, an immigrant's adjustment to America, and the human drama behind the scenes of an internist's office. We met extraordinary people who changed our lives forever, and I have nothing but respect for them. I have used their language in places for authenticity, not scorn. I have deliberately distorted events and places and names to protect identities. The characters are remixed and recreated so as to provide individual privacy, while sharing the overall experience.

As a physician, I witness much suffering and pain, but the compassion and decency of patients and friends always radiates through and strengthens me. My family and I are often overcome with the affection we have received from them. I hope this book conveys the love and gratitude we feel toward them.

—Sandip V. Mathur, MD

CHAPTER ONE

Stung

"Doc, this is Ben Grimes, in the ER. We got incoming! You on call?"

"Yes."

"Where's Doc Becker?"

"He's gone to Dallas for a wedding."

"Doc Bulent or Doc Faraday in town?"

"No. I don't know where they are, but Dr. Becker told me they were out of town this weekend."

There was a pause.

"The family *wanted* Doc Becker."

"I told you, he's not here. There is no other doctor in town, just me."

"Just you? You're the new young doc, right?"

"Right! So what's up?"

He sighed.

"Tommy Two-Ton's on his way to the ER. He looks bad!"

"Who's Tommy? What happened?"

"Local boy, Tommy. Tommy Teegarten. Rancher. Whose daddy and baby brother died in that car wreck last week?"

"No, I didn't know that. I just got here yesterday."

"Yesterday! Boy, you got thrown in the deep end, Doc!"

"Guess so."

"Him and his mamma only ones left, Doc, so his mamma wants Doc Becker."

I was irritated.

"I told you, he's *not here*. He's out of town!"

"And you're the only doc in the county? You mind if I put in a call for Doc Becker? Maybe he's somewhere close."

"Go ahead. What's the problem with Tommy?"

"He's allergic to bee stings. Got stung at the cemetery. Stung a *bunch*!"

"How are his vital signs?"

"Stable for now, but he doesn't look good. You want me to call you as soon he gets here? In case I can't get hold of Doc Becker?"

I had seen a similar case in London. A young man had been stung on his neck and had choked rapidly. We had struggled to save him, and the memory set alarm bells ringing.

"No, I'm coming right away. Get the crash cart ready! Call lab and X-ray and get the respiratory tech! Tommy can die from that!"

Within ten minutes, I was in the ER. I swung off Pecan Street and parked in the first spot. The hospital was an old reddish-black building, two floors tall. The entrance to the ER was a ramp, and the ER itself was a faded, prefabricated unit jammed on the side facing the parking lot. It was dusk; the ambulance stood reversed at the base of the ramp, and three paramedics heaved Tommy up. One also clamped an oxygen mask over his face, and the other two held him down. A fourth scampered alongside holding up a bag of saline with an IV line bobbing down to his elbow. They slammed past the double doors at the top of the ramp and charged inside, and I ran in right after them.

One look at Tommy and I felt a familiar knot in my stomach. He rattled around on the gurney, and arched and caved as he sucked air in and pushed it out with difficulty, flushed and bloated, gasping and gurgling. He was big, over six feet and at least two hundred and fifty pounds, stripped, and drenched in sweat. I was filled with dread.

He looks terrible, I thought. *He looks like the others before they crashed and died! The allergic reaction is causing swelling and obstruction of his airway. He could choke to death in minutes right in front of me. On my first day? This can't be happening!*

The paramedics swarmed over him, rolling him around on the gurney, replacing leads, and slipping on a hospital gown. I was experienced in emergency resuscitations and had done at least a hundred over my nine years as a doctor, often as the leader of the crash team. But they had all been in big teaching hospitals in London and Houston, and I always had access to specialists to back me up.

Calm down, I reassured myself. *You've done this many times.*

I glanced around quickly. I stood in a small rectangular room, about fifteen feet by thirty feet, painted or turning yellow. A sagging ceiling supported an operating room light, whose folded arm wobbled overhead. An array of low glass cupboards lined the short side of the room,

4

and their tops doubled as a writing desk and a filing area. The adjacent long side had a small window, which admitted the only natural light into the operating room. Next to the window, a feeble air conditioner coughed and hacked fitfully. I looked out; the parking lot was unpaved, and several trucks swung in, swerving past the ambulance and raising clouds of dust. A crowd gathered and framed the ambulance, and faces turned toward the window.

I turned and looked at Ben Grimes. He was tall, easily over six feet, and had a bald, bullet-shaped head. His eyes were slits, and he sported a thin moustache that continued vertically down at both ends. He was tanned and well built, had a *Semper Fi* tattoo on his left arm and a military bearing. Ben resembled an oxygen cylinder.

"Y'all, hurry up and get outta the way!" Ben shouted. "Doc's gotta check Tommy!"

Within seconds, the room cleared and only a nurse and a paramedic remained. A hush fell. They looked at me.

Do something! I thought.

It seemed too quiet to be the prelude to death. The monitor said it all: a rapid heart rate, low blood pressure, and dropping oxygen level. The nurse and paramedic wiped his chest, slapped on leads, fastened an oxygen mask, started an intravenous drip, then bundled up his clothes, which were drenched with sweat and urine, and hurled them into a corner. Tommy retched loudly, rolled on his side, and vomited. We recoiled, then swabbed him quickly, wiping his face and chest clean again. The room reeked sharply of rotten meat.

"Suction him! Reverse Trendelenberg position!" I ordered, and they tilted the bed so his head was higher than his feet. This reduced the risk of stomach contents getting sucked into his lungs.

"Almost ready, Doc!" Ben announced. "Getting the crash cart and calling in the lab tech an' respiratory tech!"

Tommy fumbled for my hand and croaked.

"Doc, am real allergic t' beestings. Buncha bees got me good, jes outside th' cemetery. Maw said, son, go to th' ER. Waited bout a half hour inside mah truck, waitin' fo' her to show up."

"You waited half an hour?"

"Know ah shunt have, but ah did. Ma eyes swelled, couldn't see right. Ma lips swelt up, Doc. Thass when ah knew et was goin' t'be bad."

I examined him. He was a big man, writhing, wider than the gurney. His blue eyes squinted in the middle of a ruddy, unshaven face. He had thick blond hair, matted with dirt. The dirt on his face and arms had fault lines, and he was pungent with sweat. The hospital gown barely covered him. His enormous belly shook, and his swollen legs stuck out over the gurney at awkward angles. In the middle of my exam, his breathing became irregular and his speech faltered. He stopped moving. *Bad sign*, I thought. *He's exhausted. He needs to make a conscious effort to keep breathing.*

I glanced at the monitor.

"Why isn't there an oxygen level?"

No one answered.

I picked up one of his spade-like hands and looked at the oximeter that was supposed to be measuring his oxygen level. His fingers and nails were coated with mud and tar.

"We have to get the tar off! The oximeter can't read his oxygen level properly if the nails are too dark!"

"We tried scrapin' it off with a knife!"

"What?"

"Pocketknife!"

"Try nail polish remover or rubbing alcohol."

"Tried it. Don't work."

"Okay, clip it on his earlobe. Those fingernails are too dirty."

"Ah was puttin' in posts round the graveyard," Tommy mumbled. "Ain't always dirty."

I nodded and lifted his wrist.

"His pulse is weak and irregular!"

"It was steady when he came in, Doc!"

"Change the leads, now! I want a new large bore IV, and give him normal saline, wide open! Send the labs stat!"

The monitor showed the heart rate slowing down. In seconds it was down to thirty beats a minute. Long, flat, green lines appeared between the spiky complexes that indicated heart contractions.

"Ah feel . . . kinda weird, Doc," Tommy gasped, then threw his head back and froze.

I grabbed his wrist but wasn't able to feel the radial pulse, so I felt in the neck to the side of the airway for the carotid artery. It was weak, but still pulsating.

"He's still got a pulse! Bradycardia! Get me some atropine now! Open those fluids! Wide open!"

I struggled to control my pitch.

I gave him the atropine and watched intently. The heart rate picked up slowly and struggled to forty-five a minute. After a few seconds, his heart rate and his breathing started to slow down again.

"Give me another atropine. He's not responding! Get me his labs. We need a blood gas; call the respiratory tech now."

Tommy had become unresponsive. He would not answer to his name and could not open his eyes or obey other commands. However, he still moaned slightly when I pinched his skin.

"At least he's still responding to pain! Call the hospital in Abilene! I need to move him there now! He needs an ICU, not a small country hospital! He needs a stat chest X-ray, portable! Tell Joe, come now! *Right now!*"

There was a burst of activity. Ben speedily changed the IV fluids, printed the heart rhythm, and ran to the lab. The respiratory technician drew blood from an artery for the blood gas analysis, and the X-ray technician squeezed his machine into the room for a chest X-ray. Anxious family members broke in repeatedly but were restrained and sent back to the waiting room. Several stood at the door, gawking and muttering. There were three men in overalls, mumbling and holding their hats in their hands, and a woman in a black pantsuit talking into a cellphone and covering her mouth with the other hand. They looked at me suspiciously.

Ben waved and cried out, "Be quiet!"

For a few seconds, the room was silent except for the wheezing of the air conditioner and the beeping of the monitor. I listened to his heart and his lungs. Tommy breathed irregularly and loudly. Then, suddenly, everyone was talking again. The respiratory therapist struggled to give Tommy a breathing treatment with nebulized albuterol, urging him to take deep breaths, while clamping a plastic mask over his nose and mouth. The nurses tried to talk to him as they examined his other arm for another IV site. I kept talking to him, but he didn't respond and didn't struggle—another bad sign. I pinched his skin again. No response now.

"What's his blood pressure?"

"Seventy systolic."

"Still got a pulse?"

"Barely. Real weak, Doc."

The family couldn't hold back and started commenting loudly.

"He looks bad, Doc!"

"Ah don't think he's gonna make it, Doc!"

"Feet's lookin' awful gray, Doc!"

"Yes, I know."

"Wish Doc Becker was here!"

Ben pushed them out and turned to me.

"Sats now eighty percent!"

"Is he on a hundred percent oxygen?"

"Yes sir!"

My mind raced. He was barely hanging on. His oxygen level was very low, and he was about to have a cardiac arrest. A sharp voice called out.

"Hey Doc! You ain't scared, are you? Doc Becker ain't in town, far's I know, so it's just you!"

I looked up. The men in overalls had retreated and a short scrawny man with an enormous handlebar moustache stood there, thoughtfully stroking his chin.

"I'm Tommy's uncle!"

"Nice to meet you."

"Hell, he looks sicker'n a dog!"

"Yes, I know."

"You on your own!"

"I know."

"Doc Becker, he really knows how t'handle these things."

"Yeah, I'll bet."

I suppressed a surge of irritation. I tried to focus. One of the men in overalls tapped Handlebar on the shoulder and whispered. Handlebar whipped out a cell phone.

"Doc *Becker* is Tommy's regular Doc!"

The man at the door asked Handlebar, "Want me try callin' him again?"

Before I could answer, Tommy stopped breathing completely and went limp. His cardiac monitor showed a brief burst of ventricular tachycardia, a very irregular heart rhythm, and then returned to a very slow rhythm.

"*Shit!* He had a run o' vee tach, Doc!"

"I know. Give him a hundred mg of lidocaine. Get me an endotracheal tube now! And clear the space near his head! I need to intubate him! Get the ventilator down, we need it here. And epi! Give me some epi now!"

I injected the lidocaine and watched for a few seconds. No further rapid bursts of the irregular contractions called ventricular tachycardia or "v-tach." I could not feel his pulse. I injected ten milliliters of "epi," or epinephrine, better known as adrenaline, and injected saline to flush it through quickly. A weak pulse returned! It remained slow, but I was relieved that it was back. I kept my finger on the carotid artery in his neck and jerked away the headboard of the bed with the other hand. Unlocking the bed, I pushed it down into the middle of the room so that I could straddle the top. I dropped to my knees, threw his pillow on the floor, and lifted the back of his neck with my left hand. His mouth flopped open. I grabbed his jaw and yanked it upward and outward, pulling his mouth wide open. His fleshy neck felt heavy and grew heavier by the second. I wanted to look straight down his throat, past his tongue and soft palate and epiglottis, at his airway.

I have to get a breathing tube in there immediately, I thought, *but I can't see the opening!*

Inside, thick beefy layers of tissue were glued together with sticky saliva and flecks of tobacco. I shook his neck in frustration and rotated it. No better.

"Suction! I need suction!"

The nurse scrambled, and handed it to me. I suctioned as much I could.

"What size ET tube, Doc?"

"He's going to need an eight. I want the Mackintosh and a stiff guide wire, a stilette."

I pushed a bunched-up towel underneath his neck and upper shoulders to allow his head to extend backward, as if he were arching his head back to look at me. I pulled the pillow on the ground under my knees and leaned forward. I suctioned his mouth clear of secretions again and pulled on sterile gloves. The nurse handed me the Mackintosh forceps and the intubating tube. I crouched and twisted myself so that I was able to look directly into his mouth and gently placed the flat blade of the instrument on Tommy's limp tongue. He did not resist at all, another bad sign. Using my left hand, I lifted the tongue and soft tissue out of the way with the blade of the forceps, and the vocal cords came into view briefly. I had to lift with enormous force to keep the jaw elevated and the tongue pushed aside. Within seconds, my hand and forearm were aching and trembling.

"Give me some cricoid pressure!"

The nurse applied pressure to the front of the neck, and I lifted the forceps again, outward and upward, with greater power. The vocal cords popped into view and stayed there. I tweaked the tip of the plastic endotracheal tube and grasped it with my right hand. Without thinking any more, I thrust it like a harpoon down past the drawn white curtains that were the vocal cords and plunged it into the trachea. I held my breath and felt the tube slide deeply into the airway. Immediately, a huge wave of satisfaction and relief swept over me. Tommy shuddered several times and became agitated. He tried to roll but was easily held down by the nurses.

"Do you think you got in, Doc?"

"I think so. Listen for breath sounds in both lungs."

I connected the endotracheal tube to a large purple oxygen bag and squeezed it to pump the oxygen deep into his lungs. I gave him a few quick breaths to saturate his lungs and pull out the trapped gases. The exhaled air was reassuringly moist, forming a film on the plastic tubing. Ben listened to the lungs, making sure he heard air enter both lungs as I squeezed the bag.

"You're in, Doc! Well done!"

I allowed myself a weak smile. It was always a challenge. Sometimes the intubation went well, but sometimes it was disastrous. I had been lucky; rather, Tommy had been lucky. I injected air into the cuff that anchored the tip of the tube in the trachea. I tugged gently. *Okay, it's secure.*

"Here's the chest film!"

The technician jammed the wet film on the viewing box. Both lungs were covered with fluffy white shadows. Areas that should have been dark and full of air were white, full of fluid leaking from his blood vessels.

"You think he's got pneumonia, Doc?"

"No. Both lungs are affected. If it was pneumonia it would be one-sided, usually."

"But he could have double pneumonia, Doc!"

"He could. *Possible*, but not *probable*."

"What?"

"Both lungs have light, fluffy white patches all over. Pneumonia is usually dense and restricted to the lobes. But the main thing is the whole clinical picture. He's got bilateral infiltrates."

"His oxygen sats have come up, though not a hundred percent sats."

I examined the edges of the lung fields on the X-ray. There was little air in the lungs; the dark areas indicating aeration were restricted to the center of the chest and fluffy white shadows filled in the rest.

"He's got *extensive* bilateral infiltrates, all the way to the periphery of the lung fields. This is bad. He has ARDS. Get me the ICU in Abilene, now!"

"What's ARDS, Doc?" asked the nurse, dialing.

"Adult Respiratory Distress Syndrome," I explained. "Happens when the blood vessels of the lungs become severely irritated and leak lots of fluid into the lungs. Tommy can't breathe because of all that fluid in his lungs. It won't let him get oxygen. It's something like drowning."

I ordered intravenous furosemide, a diuretic, and hydrocortisone, a steroid. I also gave intravenous Benadryl, an antihistamine. Tommy's body shuddered and started moving again. He suddenly struck out at the respiratory technician, who jumped out of the way. He hit the IV pole instead and it came crashing down. The tubing was jerked out, and blood and saline sprayed the floor.

"His IV is out! His IV is out! Hold him down, we need to start another one, right now!"

"Let's give him two milligrams of Versed to calm him down," I decided, "and try the IV in the other arm."

They had just started the second IV line when Tommy started bucking again. He almost pulled out the new line. The paramedics scuttled into the room.

"We're ready for him, Doc. Chopper ain't comin', so we gonna take him by ambulance. I just gotta get the handover from the ER nurse. Is it Ben?"

"Yes, but you can't take him like this! I'm going to give him another two of Versed. And I am going to stitch that IV in place. How are his vitals now?"

"Blood pressure ninety-eight over fifty-eight, pulse one hundred and fifteen."

"Give me some four-o silk for stitching."

I injected a little lidocaine first and numbed the skin around the IV site, then used the curved needle to take a few bites of skin and draw the needle and thread through the perforations on the side flanges of the IV tubing. In a few minutes, it was secured.

"Just need a list of his meds, Doc."

"Get it from Ben, I guess. Almost done."

A squeaky voice pierced the air.

"Doc! Doc, I'm his mother!"

I turned around. A stout lady stood behind me, framed by a clutch of family members. She was short and had a square face with gray hair and twitching eyes. She opened and closed her mouth several times before saying anything more. She had been standing there for a while, as no one seemed to have moved back. I hoped I hadn't said anything negative. She stepped forward and grasped my hand.

"Is he gonna be awright?"

I looked back at Tommy. He was stretched out, naked again, his meager hospital gown pulled up and bunched on his chest. He was intubated and connected to a ventilator, sported a bloody bandage on one arm and an IV stitched in on the other. He was connected to a heart monitor and had a blood pressure cuff on his right leg. There was a sea of discarded vials, boxes, paper, alcohol wipes, needle casings, heart recordings, and used tubing on the floor. The ventilator honked and blew authoritatively and flashed its messages in green semaphore. Ben jumped forward and threw a towel over his loins. He spoke up.

"Well, we've stabilized him, ma'am. He is still very sick. But we are going to send him to Abilene and admit him to the ICU there."

She looked unconvinced. Ben reiterated.

"Ma'am, he was very sick but he's okay for now. He's going to be fine."

Tommy moaned loudly and lurched to one side. Ben sprang to his side and yelped, "Whoa!"

"There's nothing to worry about, ma'am," I said. I tried to sound calm.

Tommy reared. Ben yelled and cursed, "Oh, *shit!*"

I spun around. Tommy tried to sit up. He had pulled a hand loose and tugged at the tube in his mouth. With a shudder, he wrenched it out, spraying Ben and a paramedic with blood and phlegm. Ben called for help and wrestled him back down. The monitor burst into angry alarms and then went silent as the leads got pulled off.

"Get the paramedics in here!"

Tommy's mother stood paralyzed, her mouth gaping.

"Ma'am, you need to go wait outside. You all need to go outside!" Ben cried.

She stood there, riveted. No one moved.

"Get me another ET tube!"

"Size eight?"

"Yes, yes!"

I drew up two milligrams of Versed and injected it. I was thankful that I had stitched in one of the IV lines; we still had access to his bloodstream. Tommy bucked and arched violently, and Ben and I held him down. He arched again, stiffened, and went limp. Within minutes, the monitor's furious staccato settled down to a steady cadence, and we heard Tommy's breath sounds slow down and become long and deep rather than rapid and shallow. Tommy calmed down gradually. We reconnected the leads and checked his blood pressure. The alarms started going off immediately.

"Doc, oxygen sats seventy-eight percent!"

"I know! I need to re-intubate him!"

"He ain't gonna letcha!"

"I know. I'm going to give him some more Versed."

"But he don't look like he's gonna make—"

Ben stopped. Tommy's mother was cradling his feet and crying softly. She bent forward and touched her forehead to his toes, then kissed them, holding on to them and squeezing them and resting her head on them. Ben turned away and remained silent. I injected another two milligrams of Versed, and Tommy went utterly limp. His head flopped backward. I pulled on protective glasses and thrust a towel under his neck again and pulled his jaw, opening his mouth wide. It was full of red froth.

"Suction! Give me suction!"

I cleared the mouth as much as possible. The oxygen monitor's alarms were getting louder and faster. I used the Mackintosh blade and tried to reinsert the tube, but his throat filled up again with blood and froth. I swore and changed to suction and looked again. It was a mess of traumatized bleeding tissue. I peered in the general direction of the vocal cords and decided to try blindly. Tommy suddenly hacked, showering my face and shirt with blood. I jumped up and dropped the tube on the floor. I felt shocked, angry, and frustrated. Handlebar stepped forward.

"Well, if *you* can't do it, better get Doc Becker. *He's* an expert!"

Handlebar had returned and stood next to Tommy's mother, an arm on her shoulder. Tommy's mother, her face now red and swollen, was about to burst into tears. Handlebar stabbed a satellite phone furiously.

"Give me another eight ET tube."

I wiped my face and set to it again. Two minutes had gone by, I reckoned. Four minutes without oxygen causes irreversible brain injury. Two minutes left. I grabbed a piece of gauze and wiped Tommy's mouth, then suctioned again. I used the Mackintosh and pulled hard, contorting my neck, trying to visualize the vocal cords.

"I got Doc Becker's number! He ain't picking up! I guess he's out of range! Seems you can't fix Tommy, we *got* to get Becker!"

I clenched my teeth and snatched the proffered ET tube. Handlebar brandished a cell phone the size of a brick in my face.

"*You* want to call him? Bet you don't want Tommy to *die!*"

His mother wailed.

One minute left! There's no time!

I cleared my mind. I looked at the twelve o'clock position in Tommy's throat and swabbed it deliberately, wiping away the mucus and clots. Handlebar swore.

"Terrible reception here! I'm steppin' out!"

The lower end of the vocal cords came into view, then vanished. I dropped the gauze and suction, and waited a few seconds with the tube. Nothing happened.

"Press down on his throat! Give me some cricoid pressure!"

The vocal cords burst out of the darkness. I whooped and plunged the beveled tip of the ET tube in, past the vocal cords, and deeply into the trachea.

"I'm in! *I'm in!*"

Tommy's mother looked puzzled. She glanced at the nurse.

"Thank you, *Jesus!*" Ben whooped.

"Give me a ten cc syringe, I need to blow up the cuff. Listen over the chest for breath sounds."

He listened and confirmed the presence of breath sounds on both sides. He gave me a thumbs-up. Handlebar came bounding in.

"Doc Becker is on his way!"

Ben stepped forward.

"We don't need him! Doc Mathur fixed him up!"

Handlebar was crestfallen. I cleaned up quickly. The monitor was chirping happily, Tommy's pulse and blood pressure were stable, and his oxygen level was 97 percent. I wanted to say something sharp to Handlebar, something sarcastic, something scathing, but I couldn't do it. Handlebar stood silently, his mouth half open. Before I could say anything, he left the room. Tommy's mother wiped her son's face and stood back and grasped his feet again.

I gave Tommy another milligram of Versed and helped move him onto a mobile stretcher. He had a good IV line, stitched in, and had a good airway. I walked with the paramedics as they wheeled him out and loaded him into the ambulance. His mother tugged my sleeve.

"Can I go with him in the ambulance?"

"I don't think so, ma'am."

She slumped but hung on.

"I can ask the paramedics, though."

I turned.

"Doc, generally we don't but this here's my aunt! So we're going to make an exemption. Sure you can come, Aunt Elaine, but you gotta get your own ride back. Can't wait."

"Ain't plannin' to come back, least, not tonight."

The ambulance had pulled up to the ramp and we managed to get him in without losing the IV or the endotracheal tube. A paramedic hooked the bag of saline to the wall. The ventilator was placed at his feet and strapped in securely. His mother clambered in and resumed her position at his feet, massaging the soles and squeezing them and humming, and kissing his toes one by one.

"You may need to give him some more sedation. Give him a little more Versed. Maybe another two milligrams."

"Okay, Doc! Will do! We'll call you if we have problems! Ten-four!"

The ambulance turned on all its wattage. Lights blazing, alarms blaring, tires squealing, it lurched out of the hospital parking lot and swerved hard to avoid the massed oxygen cylinders and the sign that said NO SMOKING. I stood in the parking lot, alone. I breathed easier, then realized that my back ached, my head throbbed, and my hands still trembled. My face was spotted with dried blood and phlegm. I thought about what had just happened, but it was too much. I headed to my car and sat inside, then remembered there was paperwork to be done. I checked my phone. Four missed calls: two from home and two from West Texas Cablevision. I called home and headed back wearily. It was a mandate of the system: you had to document everything. If it wasn't documented, it hadn't really happened.

Ben was cleaning up, and a janitor had appeared. Ben clapped me on the back and thrust a clipboard and a bundle of paper at me.

"Here ya go! Ain't over till the paperwork's over!"

I nodded grimly and set to work. Ben returned. He handed me a card.

"Oh, almos' forgot. His uncle left this for you."

"The guy with the big handlebar moustache?"

"Yep. That's him."

I sat down, wrote everything out in as much detail as possible, and dictated my notes. I reviewed the EKG recordings and the lab reports. I had the nurse fax my handwritten notes and all the lab results to the ICU in Abilene. Finally, it was all over. I thanked Ben and stepped out into the parking lot and looked at my Corolla, covered in white dust. The other trucks had gone, following the ambulance to Abilene. I reached in my pocket for something to wipe the windscreen. I found only Handlebar's business card and bit on it as I wiped the glass with both hands. I sat down inside and glanced at the card. Handlebar's business card read:

JAMES WENTWORTH TEEGARTEN,
DISTRICT ATTORNEY.

CHAPTER TWO

The Cable Guy

The doorbell rang early the next morning.

"The doorbell? Who could it be this early? It's *Sunday!*" Maya groaned. The doorbell rang out again, and her cellphone started chirping. She tumbled out and rummaged in her purse. I scrambled in pajamas to the front door, glancing into the girls' room. They were still asleep.

There was a lanky fellow at the door, in jeans and denim shirt that announced *Ronnie*. He took off his cap and extended his hand amicably.

"Morning, Doc! How are ya this morning?"

"I'm fine. Who are you?"

"I'm Ronnie with Cablevision, your cable provider."

"The cable company?"

"Yes sir! At your service!"

"What are you doing here this early?"

"I need to see your cable box so I can activate your service."

I looked at him, confused.

"I left a couple of messages for you yesterday, sir. Did you check your messages?"

I remembered the two missed calls.

"What are you doing here at seven a.m. on a Sunday morning?"

He grinned and stepped back, and waved a hand at the neighboring houses, all single-level, neat brick rectangles with clipped grass, holly bushes, and oak trees. The Stars and Stripes fluttered in front of two of them, applauding the dewy silence of morning.

"Doc, I'm the cable guy for this entire county. Folks here love their cable! I got no spare time in the week. This is special, just for you. You following the OJ Simpson trial?"

"Who isn't?"

"Yeah, that's the truth. Millions of people watching. Trial of the century. Got to have your cable!"

"Did you try to call me yesterday?"

"Yeah. I heard you was in the ER; you saved Tommy Two-Ton. Figured I'd say thanks by helpin' you out some before church."

"Why do you need me?"

"I ain't permitted on your property without your permission. You could shoot me if I was just walkin' around your backyard, on account of ownership law!"

"Actually, I'm not the owner."

"I know. Ed Dunlap be the owner. How much rent you paying?"

I looked at him in surprise.

"That's okay if you don't want to tell. Word is, you pay seven hundred a month, but that's robbery to me. You ready?"

"For what?"

"Come with me to your cable box. I know where it is, it's in the back between your garage and the house."

I hesitated, then went back inside and reassured Maya. I pulled on a jacket, picked up the keys from their perch behind the door, and stepped outside again. My daughters, Priya and Anjali, had woken up and followed me outside in their pajamas. They pushed back their hair, rubbed their eyes, and looked up at the two of us. Priya ran back inside and reappeared with her cowgirl boots on. Anjali grabbed my leg and gazed at the stranger. Ronnie beamed.

"Well, now! Who do we have here?"

The girls smiled shyly.

"The older one is Priya and she's five, and the younger one's Anjali and she's two."

"They're real pretty! Two beautiful little girls!"

"Thank you. Anjali, please put on your slippers if you want to come outside. Priya already has her boots on."

Anjali shook her head. Anjali had an almond-shaped face, bangs, and pouty lips. She spoke very little. My daughter twisted and buried her face behind my knee, then peeked out.

"No."

"You need to. You might step on a thorn. You don't want to step on a thorn, do you?"

"No!"

I opened the door wide for her to go back inside.

"Hurry up! Get your slippers."

Anjali shook her head vigorously. She detached herself and raised her arms.

"Carry me!"

"No, get your slippers!"

"No, you carry me!"

"Whoa! She's made up her mind, Doc!"

"Anjali!"

It was no use. I hoisted her onto my shoulders and closed the door. I crouched to lock it.

"You don't need to lock your door, Doc! This is Hotspur!"

"It's a habit."

"Doc, in Hotspur, most folks don't lock they homes or they cars. They never lock nothing! Me, I lock my van when it's full of stuff, got to, regulations, but when I'm home, no siree, nothing's locked!"

"It's a habit. I grew up in India, and I always locked and double-locked doors. It'll take me some time to change, I guess."

I checked the locked door.

"So, where were you before you come here?"

"Houston."

"Houston! I'm sorry!"

"Sorry?"

"Sorry you had to live in Houston. Houston's hot, dirty, crowded, sweaty. Houston is the armpit of America!"

"I've heard. I didn't mind it too much."

"Really? Where you from?"

"I was born in India. I got my medical degree in India, and most of my training in England. What about you? Born here?"

"Born here, raised here, lived here all a' my life. Texan by the grace of God!"

"Ever wanted to live in a big city?"

"Hell, no! My brother lives in Galveston, and I visit him, and no siree, not for me! You can keep them crowds and freeways and that stink of oil! I'm just an old country boy!"

He pulled a bag out of his truck parked in the driveway.

"You got any other kids?"

"Just these two." Priya looked up and beamed and Anjali lurched.

She grabbed my hair to steady herself and made me wince. I held her ankles firmly and paused as she wriggled.

"I okay now!" Anjali announced.

"Where we going, Dad?" asked Priya, skipping.

"To the backyard."

"We going to the backyard, little lady! We going to get you all set up for TV!"

"We have these two, and they're a handful!"

"Good deal! I got four, two a mine, two a hers. Gets a little rambunctious come Christmas! What's your missus do?"

"She's an architect."

"Architect! Whoa! We got some high-class folks here, I can tell, yes sir! *Architect!*"

He paused, thought, then moved on.

"But there ain't much work for a architect in Hotspur County."

"She's busy with the girls."

"That she will be. Remember, you got to keep the missus happy! If Mama ain't happy, nobody's happy!"

"Yes, I know. So you have four kids?"

"Well, don't know if we can call 'em kids anymore. Youngest's eighteen, going on thirty. You ever been divorced?"

"No."

"Made the first one twenty-four years. Pulled it through, worked on it, just didn't work out. Tried, though."

He looked straight ahead. He swallowed and pursed his lips.

"She left me. Younger man."

We walked past the garage and he glanced inside.

"Say, what you got there, Doc?"

"Toyota Corolla, Toyota Camry."

"Toyota! You like them foreign cars?"

"I do like Toyotas, they're reliable cars."

"No, no, Doc! This is truck country! Get you a truck!"

I grinned at the thought.

"No, I'm serious! Doc, you got a serious choice to make!"

"Sedan or truck?"

"No, truck's a given. Chevy or Ford?"

"Chevy or Ford?"

"Either you're a Chevy guy or you're a Ford guy."

"What are you?"

He pulled himself up and answered gruffly.

"Chevy! My granddad had a Chevy and my dad had a Chevy and I had a Chevy since I was sixteen!"

"Since sixteen?"

"Fifteen, actually. Farmboys can get 'em early. First truck I ever did drive was my daddy's old pickup. What was your first—vehicle?"

"This is it."

"What!"

"I had a bicycle in med school and internship in India. Most of us had bicycles, so that wasn't unusual. In England I never had a car, used public transport: buses, their subway."

"Doc, this is Texas and in Texas we *drive*, we drive everywhere! You need a truck for them dirt country roads! And how you gonna hunt with a little see-dan car?"

He looked at me earnestly, then stepped back in surprise.

"You don't hunt?"

"No."

"Fish?" he ventured, hopefully.

"Not really."

"What do you *do,* Doc?"

"I like to read books and watch movies. Spend time with my family. We go biking and walking. I like to work out on my treadmill."

"I don't know, Doc. You don't hunt or shoot or fish or drive a truck. How you gonna fit in?"

We reached the gate, and I took out my keys again. Securing Anjali with one hand, I unlocked the gate with the other and swung it open. Ronnie shook his head in disbelief.

"Lord almighty! You lock your gate too?"

I shrugged. Priya rushed to her swing and kicked off. Anjali was content to stay on my shoulders and swung around, tethered tightly.

"Houston does that to you."

"Big cities, I tell ya! Big cities! So where you from, originally, Doc, England or India?"

"I'm from India originally. Like I said, I did my basic degree in India, then went to London and finished most of my training there. Then I came to Houston to specialize and go back to London, but we fell in love with Texas and wanted to stay."

"Where'd you train in Houston?"

"I did my fellowship in gastroenterology from Baylor and MD Anderson and then I had to go back and do my residency at UT."

"What's gastro . . . what you said?"

"Gastroenterology. Diseases of the stomach and intestine and colon and liver."

"So you're a specialist?"

"Yes."

"Not a family practitioner?"

"No, but I am an internist, and that's like a family practitioner. Only I don't see children or deliver babies."

"Don't see *children?* Don't deliver *babies?*"

"No. Only adults. Anyone over eighteen."

Ronnie shook his head slowly, disappointed.

"Don't hunt, don't shoot, don't fish, don't drive a truck, don't see kids, don't deliver babies. *Man!*"

"Good thing for me you weren't on the selection committee."

"So what'd you do before that? Before Houston?"

"I was in London."

"London, England?"

"Yes."

"Whoa! So you started out in India, then you went to England, then Houston, Texas, and now here in Hotspur, Texas!"

"That's right. Kind of a long journey, right?"

"You never lived in a city less than a million people?"

"No, I don't think so."

"And here you are in Hotspur, Texas, ten thousand souls in five thousand square miles!"

"And two doctors."

"Did you do your medical degree from London?"

"No, I got my medical degree in India. I went to London to get experience and training in general medicine and liver diseases."

"So why'd you come to Houston in the first place?"

"I was getting too specialized in London. I had all this training in liver diseases and liver transplantation, but no training in general regular gastroenterology. So I applied to Houston and asked for a fellowship in gastroenterology."

"And they gave you that?"

"Yes, there was an opening at that time, and they gave it to me."

"Were you thinking of going back to London after doing what extra training you needed?"

"Exactly! I thought I would finish my training in general gastroenterology and then go back to England or maybe even India."

"So what happened?"

"We both—my wife, Maya, and I—liked it here so much we didn't want to go back to England."

"Here?"

"The US. We wanted to stay in the United States."

"Someone like you, all that training, transplants, and research, you shoulda become a teacher, you know, like a professor or something."

"Actually, I did try for a teaching job at a VA hospital. They interviewed me and offered me a job."

"So how'd you end up here?"

"I interviewed here in Hotspur as well. There is a shortage of doctors here, and they also offered me a green card if I would come and practice here."

"So you chose practicing medicine in Hotspur over teaching and research and all?"

"Long story, but, yes, interviewed both places, decided to come to Hotspur."

He opened the cable box and fished inside it. He poked around with a screwdriver and grunted. He flicked a few switches, then stopped. He turned to me and asked sternly.

"Tell me, why did you *really* come here? What do you *really* want out of this place?"

I was taken aback. I studied him intently. He had a pleasant face, weathered skin, slate eyes hidden in slits, scarred lips, and a fixed smile. I looked closely, and there was no malice, nothing but curiosity in his expression. I decided to be direct.

"I'm here because I want a green card."

He thought for a minute.

"That's it?"

"Yes."

He worked on the box, nodding his head slowly. I regretted it immediately. I should have said, *I'm here because I want to start my own practice in a small town. I want to serve this community. I want to give back.* That would have sounded better. But I had been swayed by his frankness and had matched it. There was more manhood in standing by the mistake, so I said nothing and waited while he processed my response and fixed the cable box.

Abruptly, he laughed and thumped the wall.

"So you ain't a child molester or a drunk?"

"What?"

"So you ain't a child molester or a drunk? Ain't been disbarred from some other state? Running away from something? Ain't a druggie or pervert?"

"Are you *crazy?*"

He stood up and wiped his fingers on his shirt. He grinned at my discomfiture, his face relaxed. He spoke calmly.

"Doc, we get the docs who been kicked out of everywhere else. That's why they come here. Then they stay a year or two, then leave and go somewheres else."

"I'm here for three years, I have a contract."

"I don't care about contracts. I'm tickled you're here, and cause you're here for a green card, and not cause you're a child molester or pervert!"

I was speechless. He flashed me a smile.

"Hope I didn't *offend* ya?"

A child molester? A pervert?

I opened my mouth and still couldn't think of anything to say.

"Mind ya, I did check with my friends at the courthouse. No criminal record on you."

I was grateful that Priya was out of earshot and that Anjali had a hearing defect. He turned to Priya.

"Whoa, little lady! I sure do like your little white cowgirl boots! Tassels and all!"

Priya beamed and swung higher.

He walked up to her and gently lifted her off the swing and set her down.

"She got a big old skeeter bite on her elbow, Doc!"

My smile was gone. I spoke grimly.

"I'll put some vinegar on the bite. That'll help."

"Vinegar for a skeeter bite! I'll be darned! How'd you figure that out?"

I suppressed my anger.

"My grandmother told me. Did it in India all the time. Stops the stinging."

"I'll be sure to try that next time! Guess I learned something today!"

I was still seething. Ronnie bubbled on, blissfully.

"I'm all done! Now we all can get ready for church! Which church you all go to?"

"Actually, we don't go to church."

He stopped and turned to see if I was serious. I pressed on grimly.

"We don't go to church."

"You *don't* go to church?"

"No."

"Why not?"

"Because we're not Christian."

"Then what are you?"

"I was raised Hindu."

"What's that?"

"It's a different religion."

"You're, like, Jewish?" he said, hopefully.

"No, Hindu."

"So where is your church or whatever?"

"We pray at home. We have a temple in Dallas, but we prefer to pray at home."

I locked the gate slowly and deliberately. We headed back to his truck in silence with Priya skipping ahead. He got in and closed the door gravely. He was concerned.

"I don't know, Doc! You don't hunt or shoot or fish or drive a truck or see kids or deliver babies and you ain't Christian! You sure qualified and trained! We are glad to have you, but you, you're *different!* I don't know if, you know, if word gets out, going to be mighty difficult to get people to come see you."

"I understand."

"All the new docs in town, we call 'em NCPDs, New Christian Prairie Doctors. What we gonna call you?"

"Just NPD. Or how about NYPD?"

"NYPD?"

"New Young Prairie Doctor."

He grinned.

"I like it."

He kept smiling and nodding as he strapped himself in and turned the ignition on. He pointed and wagged his finger.

"Mr. NYPD, I like you. You know, I see many people that say they're Christian but have no Christian values. You say you're not Christian but you have Christian values."

I smiled.

"You know what? I think you got love in your heart."

"I like what I do. I like looking after people."

Ronnie looked ahead and spoke quietly.

"If you got love in your heart, you got Jesus in your heart."

"I'm going to do my best," I said awkwardly.

"I know. Just don't know how you gonna make it work here. Maybe this is all a big mistake. You being a specialist, professor kinda guy, city kinda guy, no truck, don't hunt, don't shoot, not even Christian."

"Well," I added weakly, "at least I'm not a child molester."

He laughed.

"Yeah, least you're not a child molester! But I don't know how you're gonna fit in here, Doc!"

He revved the engine.

"Well, Mr. NYPD, God in His wisdom surely got to have a plan for ya! I just can't figure it out, but God moves in strange and wondrous ways, His miracles to perform! Hey, Doc, I got to get to church!"

Ronnie waved and roared off. I thought about what he said and thought back. It had all happened so fast. The original plan was to go to the VA Hospital in Rochester, New York, as an assistant professor of gastroenterology. I had trained in internal medicine, specialized in gastroenterology, further specialized in liver diseases and liver transplantation, written several papers, done laboratory research. I had always imagined myself as an academician, doing more research, writing more papers, teaching students, seeing patients, and living in a big city. Maybe Ronnie was right. How *did* I end up in a small prairie town?

Strange and wondrous.

CHAPTER THREE

The Innerview

In October 1993, I had tried repeatedly to find a job as a teaching or research doctor, but had failed. I had applied to three academic centers associated with VA hospitals. Two had rejected me within days because of my visa; the third offered me the job. To my shock, Professor Wilkinson, my chief in Houston, had made them withdraw the offer. With four months left on my visa, I abandoned hopes of staying in academics and applied to several rural underserved hospitals. They needed doctors and had the ability to petition the Immigration Service for green cards as an inducement to recruit foreign-trained doctors.

The Hotspur Hospital in west central Texas responded promptly and called me for an interview. I spoke to the administrator, John Abbott, and several staff members before coming. I learnt that there were three doctors in town. Dr. Becker and Dr. Bulent were full-time and covered the emergency room. Dr. Kennedy was part-time and ran a clinic four mornings a week. Dr. Becker and Dr. Kennedy were unhappy about foreign-trained doctors, and Dr. Bulent was trying to recruit a fellow Turk, an obstetrician-gynecologist training in New York. The final decision had to be made by the hospital's governing board. I anticipated some critical questioning from them, especially given the pressure from the other doctors.

I had registered those concerns and had shown up for the interview. In the morning, I toured the hospital and was interviewed by the hospital administrator, John Abbott, and by the chief nurse, Penny Smalley. We had gotten along well. I had rested in my motel room that afternoon and prepared for the critical interview with the board at six p.m. At five-thirty, I stood in the parking lot outside the log cabin. I was early, so I wasn't surprised that there were just three trucks in the parking lot. The lot was unpaved and dusty, ringed by a rough-hewn wooden fence. A metal sign on the roof announced, simply, BONNIE'S. Everyone knew it was a steakhouse.

I wore a dark suit, white shirt, and blue tie, and carried a slim briefcase. I looked around and took it all in. Behind me, the 83/84 Highway rumbled with eighteen-wheelers, and just beyond that was the Shiloh Inn, PROUDLY OWNED BY AMERICANS, where I was staying. In front and to my right, a billboard declared HOTSPUR: OPEN FOR BUSINESS! MUNICIPAL AIRPORT, TURN RIGHT. On my left, an abandoned prefabricated building with boarded-up windows slumped under a sign that said BOOT SCOOTERS: BAR, ENTERTAINMENT AND NIGHT CLUB. A backdrop of mesquite and live oak trees loomed behind these two buildings.

The smell of barbeque and roasting meat hit like a whip. It was exhilarating! My eyes opened wide and I inhaled deeply, sucking it in and savoring. I could smell mesquite and hickory as well, and wafts of bacon and onions with the tickle of roasting peppers.

"You must be the new doc!"

The door had been opened, and a large lady stood there. An enormous white beehive hairdo, tinged with blue, crowned her face, and a profusion of chunky jewelry hung on her ears and cascaded around her neck. She waved her hands and removed her gloves as she descended the steps. She was remarkably agile for someone so large and wearing such high heels. Her face was hidden behind a dense patina of makeup, but her blue eyes sparkled and her smile was welcoming.

"So nice to see you! I'm Bonnie Bail, th'owner of this place! You are kinda early!"

We shook hands warmly. I noticed that her fingers were studded with large rings. She smelled of barbecue and musk.

"Thank you! Well, I didn't have anything else to do so I thought I would come here and kind of get ready. For the evening."

"Oh, yeah, for the innerview. We done got the table ready, so come on in! Sit you down an' git something! Have some tea or something! Make yawself right at home, Doc! So nice to have you here!"

The innerview. I liked that.

Inside, it was smaller than I expected, and dark. There were fluorescent tubes and neon signs on the walls and multicolored Christmas lights strung up in between. Metal signs were everywhere: Budweiser Beer, Miller Light, Rasmussen's Oilfield Supply, Pepsi-Cola, Dr. Pepper

Made In Dublin 10 cents, and quips on wooden boards. One caught my eye: *I wasn't born in Texas but got here fast as I could!*

The table and chairs were all hand-carved, rough but handsome, and well-worn with use. Bonnie came back and handed me a menu.

"Don't suppose you want a beer? Maybe ice tea?"

"Ice tea would be great."

"Surely."

I sat at the middle of a long table, sipping my tea.

Bonnie came back to me and asked conspiratorially, "Hey, Doc! Would you look at this rash for me?"

She showed me her left wrist. She had a patchy red blistering rash with bumps and scratch marks. I held her wrist and rotated it. It was there on the other side as well. It went all around her wrist, like a circle.

"I got it on the other wrist's well, Doc, jes not as bad!"

A similar rash, less severe, snaked around her right wrist. I was puzzled.

"Anywhere else?"

"Little bit on my neck."

She put down her tray and lifted up her necklaces. A similar rash, with more redness and blistering, went all around her neck like a collar. *A ring-like rash around the left wrist, a lesser one around the right, and a faint rash around the neck.* Could it be an allergy to something? The jewelry? But only one of the three rashes was in contact with jewelry. Suddenly, it all made sense!

"Did you change your watch strap recently?"

She took a step back.

"How'd you know that?"

"Then it was too tight and you wore the watch on the right?"

She was shaking her head in disbelief.

"Maybe you had matching necklaces?"

She turned away, shaking her head, then turned back.

"Just how did you know all that?"

"Because I've seen it before. It's a nickel allergy. You had an allergy to nickel in your watchstrap. You wore it on the left then the right but you're not wearing it now, so it was just too tight. The strap has nickel and you are allergic to it. The necklace has a little nickel in it as well, you better stop wearing that."

She stepped back and looked at me squarely.

"You know what, Doc, that is *exactly* right!"

"I had a case just like that in London; that's how I recognized it."

"So what should I do? Go see a specialist in Abilene?"

"No, just stop wearing anything with nickel and just put a little hydrocortisone on your rash twice daily. It should go away in a week."

She smiled in delight.

"I don't have to go to a fancy specialist! You just saved me a bunch a'money!"

Then her face clouded over.

"So I'm allergic to jewelry?"

"No, just jewelry with nickel."

She thanked me and sailed away.

Slowly, the place filled up. Many came in overalls, stained and heavy with dried mud. Some were dressed formally, with bolo ties and crisp white shirts and starched jeans. Men pulled chairs back for the women and then helped adjust them as the women were seated. They addressed each other with "Ma'am" and "Sir," and most bowed their heads and said a prayer before they ate. Everyone drank iced tea and about half drank beer as well. They cast a few glances in my direction. Some looked longer, with frank curiosity. I checked my briefcase. It had some documents that I had picked up from the medical library in Houston. I placed it between my chair and the next, out of view. I took off my coat and hung it on my chair, trying to look a little casual. I kept my tie on.

The members of the hospital board showed up together, exactly on time. There were six directors, and four had come to Bonnie's that night.

"Bill Hayden, pleased t' meet you."

"Trent Garrett, how d'you do?"

"I'm Emily Youngblood and I'm delighted to meet you, doctor."

"Rusty Johnson. Call me Coach. I'm the head of the board."

We sat down. All four sat opposite me. Mrs. Youngblood stood up.

"Whoa! This looks like an inquisition! I'm going to go sit *next* to this young man!"

At first, the three men seemed ill at ease. They spoke awkwardly about the weather, the drought, and the Dallas Cowboys. Talking about sports relaxed them, and Bonnie came with pitchers of iced tea and plates of barbecue ribs.

"Well, honey, I haven't even ordered yet!" Coach protested, helping himself to a rib.

"Coach Rusty, I see you in the parking lot and I order the ribs. I know what you want!"

"Heck, no need for me to order! You know what I always order for my main course?"

"Sixteen ounce done rare, horseradish on the side."

Coach Johnson slapped his hand on the table and his face twisted with delight.

"That's me!"

―――――――

Bonnie smiled and took the orders. She explained the menu to me.

"See, Doc, most folks like the ribeye. Twelve or sixteen ounces of grade A beef. Well done means cooked hard, rare means cooked light with all natural juices flowin, real tender. Medium is kinda in between."

"I'll have the sixteen ounce, done medium."

The men nodded approvingly. Coach cleared his throat and started. He was a lean black man who spoke slowly and deliberately. The others watched him and nodded.

"See, Doc, you're here for the interview. But we done looked at your papers and you're good on paper. *On paper.* See, we got a bunch a' doctors come through here, just don't stick it out. We need a good, solid doctor. We're all good folks, straight an' honest, tell it like it is. So I'll get to the point. Maybe you, sir, are overqualified for this job."

He straightened up and crossed his arms. I regarded him from across the table and formulated my answer. I wanted to get it right. Emily Youngblood turned to look at me.

"We mean, you have training in *liver disease* and even in *transplantation*," she explained. "You're so specialized that we are concerned you won't like it here. We need a family doctor, or an internal medical doctor, a prairie doctor, not a specialist."

"I understand. Let me explain, because I have given this a lot of thought. I left London because I thought I was getting too specialized. I came to Houston to do general gastroenterology."

"What, exactly, is that?"

"Diseases of the stomach and colon and liver. It's in his resume," Bill Hayden muttered.

He was tall and well-built with a weathered face and slits for eyes. He spoke slowly, barely moving his lips.

"And, after I did my general gastroenterology training, I decided to stay in the US and applied for a Texas medical license. For that, I needed to have a residency in internal medicine. Internal medicine is the basic training and, usually, you do your specialty training *after* that. I did my specialty training *first*, at Baylor, and then went back and did my general basic medicine again so I could get my Texas medical license. So, actually, I am just finishing my *second* round of training in basic internal medicine."

"Now I'm confused," Coach Johnson interrupted. "So you did your fellowship at Baylor in your specialty—GI—without doing a residency in internal medicine?"

"That's right," I responded.

"How could they let you do that?"

"Because I had already done a residency in internal medicine in London, England. Baylor accepted my training in England as being equal to the residency training in the US. The State Board gave me a temporary medical license. But when I wanted a full license the State Board said no, you need to go back and do a residency here in the US in internal medicine."

"So after all that you went back and did a *second* round of training in basic internal medicine?" Emily Youngblood was incredulous.

"Exactly. So you see, I have trained twice in basic internal medicine, first in England and then again here in Texas. And the most recent training I have is in internal medicine."

They all looked at each other. I knew that had impressed them. Coach turned back to me and said, "So you *are* an internal medical doctor."

"First and foremost!"

"What about gastrology? I mean, your specialty?"

"I can do that too, on the side. But I'm a primary doctor first and a specialist second."

Coach Johnson shook his head and held up a hand. "We should ask Dr. Becker and Dr. Bulent and Dr. Kennedy about all this first before makin' this young man an offer."

Bill Hayden shook his head.

"Forget it, Coach. Doc Kennedy's packing his bags, he's going to Plainview to retire. And Doc Bulent and Doc Becker can't stand to be in the same room's each other, that's how come they ain't here tonight. They ain't gonna help us decide nothing!"

Coach sighed then turned back and demanded, "Bonnie! When's those steaks coming? Sometime this year?"

The steaks were superb and put everyone in a good mood. We pushed back from the table and Coach whipped out a toothpick. He attacked his molars as Emily Youngblood continued the questioning.

"What does your wife think of West Texas? Do you think she can adapt to this place?"

"Maya is very excited about the idea of moving here. She has been on the internet and has been looking at schools and house prices. She is keen to come here."

"She has no worries about moving here?"

"She is worried you don't have a Target."

They laughed.

"We got us a Walmart in Brownwood," Bill Hayden rumbled.

"She's looking after our two little girls. Houston is crazy. She wants to get out of Houston and come somewhere calm."

They looked at each other and nodded.

"She a nurse?"

"No, she's an architect. She specializes in residences. She might resume working later. But right now, she's a full-time stay-at-home mom."

"That's right. You've got two little ones. Both girls?" Coach inquired.

"Yes sir."

"Gonna try for a boy?"

"Coach!" Emily reproached.

"It's a fair question. Well, are you?"

"No, we're happy with what we have."

"I heard in India they like boys, not girls."

"In some places, that is true. But that's not our way of thinking."

"How old are your kids?"

"Five years and two years old."

"Five and two! Why, they're just barely hatched! But the five-year-old can go to kindergarten. Two-year-old's gonna be at home a long time."

"My wife, Maya, is used to the idea of being a home mom. She doesn't want to start working."

Coach Johnson folded his hands and leaned forward over his empty plate.

"Doc, we got another issue. You know that Doc Bulent and Doc Becker just don't see eye to eye. Doc Bulent says he got a couple Turkish docs in New York and he wants us to sponsor *them* instead of you. Says they his kinfolk and he can vouch for them. Husband and wife, man's internal medicine and woman's ob-gyn."

Trent Garrett leaned forward. He had white hair, parted neatly in the middle, and a white moustache, and wore a red scarf around his neck. He spoke softly and deliberately.

"You see, we never had an ob-gyn doctor interested in Hotspur. So we was thinking, hey, maybe we could get some babies born here in Hotspur. Kinda neat, having babies born in the hospital again."

He looked at Coach.

"I got to say this, I like the idea of babies bein born in this hospital," Coach agreed, nodding.

"Doc Bulent says they already have their medical licenses in New York and so they could easily get their Texas licenses!"

"Where are those two doctors right now?"

"Finishing up in New York."

I pounced.

"Let me tell you something. I've looked this up. If they are in New York, they *must* be on provisional licenses. New York is pretty strict on licensing. You can't get a full New York medical license unless you're an American citizen, and obviously they are not US citizens. They cannot get licenses to practice in Texas. Let me prove it to you."

I reached back and pulled out some documents from my briefcase and gave them to Coach and Emily Youngblood. When I had made my hotel booking, the owner, Ken Patel, had told me that two Turkish doctors from New York were going to be interviewed the following week. I had come prepared.

"I just have two copies, but as you can see, they are from the Medical Register, which records all rules about medical licensing in the United States. Look at the column for New York."

"It says, US citizenship required for full licensure, just what you said."

The others took the papers and scanned them, nodded, and handed them back.

"New York will *not* grant them full medical licenses, because they aren't US citizens. They are in training and are on provisional licenses.

You can only get a Texas medical license by reciprocity if you have a *full* medical license in the other state."

"So you're saying that they would not be able to get Texas medical licenses?" Coach asked.

"Exactly."

"What if they got a full license in another state?" Trent Garrett wondered.

"It would take months to years to get a full license in another state. Then it takes at least six months, often longer, much longer, for someone coming from out of state to get a Texas license by reciprocity. If you qualified overseas, then it can take even longer. They have to verify everything from your medical school so they send letters to every medical school and hospital you worked at, and it takes a *long* time for all the documents to be returned and checked. And that's if you have a full medical license in another state, and they can't have full New York licenses because they're not US citizens. So they are not eligible for Texas licenses."

Coach looked at me squarely.

"You already have your Texas license?"

"Yes, sir."

"Full and unrestricted?"

"Yes, sir."

He looked at the others. He picked up a toothpick and chewed it. Trent Garrett played with the salt shaker. I held my breath. Bill Hayden finally spoke.

"Seems t'me we need a doc sooner than later."

"Bird inna han' worth two inna bush, Coach!" Trent agreed.

Emily Youngblood hesitated. I turned to look at her. She was petite, had short white hair and a perky nose. She gazed at me intently.

"Dr. Mathur, I just wonder if you are doing all this just because you are so keen to stay in the United States and not because you want to have a medical practice in Hotspur."

Immediately, I had their complete attention.

"I've thought about that. I intend to start my medical practice and I love Texas. Starting a practice in Hotspur instead of Houston is going to be different, but I would have the hospital's backing for a year and the hospital would help me with an income guarantee for a year. I couldn't get any help like that in Houston. I realize that starting a practice in a small town has its own challenges, but I am sure I can handle it. I have all the training I need and I'm ready to go to work!"

"Doc, what do you like about Texas? Why not Beverly Hills or DC or something else?"

"Trent, I'm from India. I like the sun. I like the people; they're like the Punjabi people I grew up with. They're straight and decent and tell it like it is. I like that. *We* like that. We love the openness. We want to live where we feel comfortable."

Bill Hayden leaned forward.

"Ah get that. We all get that. But Texas ain't India an' it ain't London. All'a folks here, born and raised here. No offence, but they might say, he ain't from here. He's a *foreigner!* What you gonna tell 'em, Doc? What you gonna tell 'em, hey?"

Coach pushed back from the table and stared down at me. I thought furiously. *What do I say?* I scanned the walls for a cue.

"I'm going to tell them, *I'm not from Texas, but I got here fast as I could!*"

They loved that. They threw their heads back and roared, and Emily Youngblood smiled from then on.

"I read that on the wall here," I admitted sheepishly.

"Course we know. Just the way you says it!"

The merriment died down, and we ordered dessert. It was pecan pie with ice cream, and we washed it down with coffee. Emily Youngblood turned to me.

"Dr. Mathur, I'm still curious. I want to know if you would be a good fit. For us, for Hotspur. For this country."

"What's your question?"

"You have two little girls?"

"Yes."

She hesitated.

"Would you let them go to public schools here or homeschool them?"

"We would send them to public schools. We would teach them at home too, of course, but we want to use public schools."

"You would let them have friends in school and let them have play dates and sleepovers? You know, where the kids spend the night at the other kid's house?"

"Sure."

"You would be okay if your girls were friendly with the boys as well as the girls?"

"Yes, of course."

"Would you be okay if they had boyfriends? White boyfriends? Black boyfriends?"

I smiled. I had thought about this many times and my grandmother had weighed in on this. She had grown up in British India and she knew all about prejudice. I was sure of my answer.

"Yes, so long as he's open-minded. The British ruled us for over a hundred years and we learnt that color and character are two different things."

"What if one of your daughters wanted to date a local boy? Would you object? Would you prefer to have them marry someone from India?"

"I believe that we are all the same. I would want the man to be a good man, honest and kind and sincere, but I don't care if he's white or brown or black or whatever. And if we are living in Texas, I think the odds are that our girls will find husbands that grew up in Texas."

Coach leaned forward and looked closely.

"Doc, the whole deal 'bout this here innerview is to see if you would be a good fit. We don't want to make another mistake. See, we're all elected by the people of Hotspur County to serve on the board an' so we got a duty. *Duty!* Duty to get our hospital running again. I'm a straight man and so I'm telling you: I have a good feeling about you. I think you *would* be a good fit."

"Thank you."

"This town ain't perfect, Doc. Nobody's perfect, no place is perfect. Used to be racist, now look at me! Black! The people here, they're good and simple people. Their forefathers had slaves, and my forefathers were those slaves, Doc! But I ain't bitter! No, sir! But what I am trying to say is this: it's not goin' to be easy to adjust."

"Coach, I've faced problems all my life. I grew up in India, struggled to get into medical school, struggled to get to England, and now I'm struggling to get this job. I know what struggling is all about. I can struggle, and I can make it work!"

"You just want this job just because you want to stay in the US?"

I paused.

"You know, my boss told me I should go back. My other professors told me there wasn't an opening for me. But I see an opportunity right here!"

"Did you know that your Professor Wilkinson sent us a letter?" Bill Hayden spoke, quietly.

He pulled out a folded paper. I was stunned.

"*What?*"

"My son-in-law works at MD Anderson and knows Prof. Wilkinson."

"We—Professor Wilkinson and I—didn't always get along."

"Prof. Wilkinson sent us a letter. He was not supportive. He says you should go back to India."

I was at a loss.

"I can explain, but it's so petty that I don't know if you'll believe me."

"Try me," Bill Hayden said.

"I was presenting a case to a bunch of medical students and Professor Wilkinson was sitting in the front row. It was about a patient who had a growth on the liver. He interrupted me halfway because he wanted to know the result of a blood test that would have made the diagnosis. But the professor in charge of the presentation told me not to announce that result and go on with the case for the sake of the medical students who needed to learn the whole approach. So I didn't give him the result. I was polite. He was angry maybe because he thought I had disobeyed him in front of the medical students."

"The other professor told you not to give out that result right away?" Coach Johnson asked.

"Yes, the professor in charge of the presentation, who was on the stage with me."

"That's it? He got upset with you over that?"

"Yes."

Bill Hayden slipped on glasses and began to read

"Doc, he said—"

Coach interrupted.

"Bill, I don't care what he said. I know something about being pushed around. I don't care to be told what to do and where to live, that's what I say. Doc, I call this the innerview. You must have an inner voice. What does your inner voice say? Stay or go back?"

"I say all your forefathers came here to this county looking for opportunity to help their families live a better life. So do I. I want a better life for my family. I have a problem with someone who tells me and my family where we should go and live. I want a better life for my family, *that's* what I want. I *like* being a doctor. I'm good at it! I'll work hard for the folks here and all of us will win."

Coach watched me curiously, then spoke.

"So you proposing we should say no to our own Dr. Bulent on the grounds that his friends can't get Texas licenses and say yes to you?"

"Yes."

"Because your inner voice says you are going to leave the high-flyin' research and the DNA and the RNA and the lab work and all behind and work with the *real* problems of *real* people in the *real* world?"

"Yes, sir."

Coach exhaled. He looked at the others. They nodded.

"I'm gonna propose to the board that we send you a contract. Mind you, I ain't promisin' you, just saying I will recommend you. Emily, when's the next meetin'?"

"Next Thursday."

"You have just met most of the board. You know Bonnie's on the board? She likes you already. Allergic to *jewelry*? What *will* that woman do? Lord Almighty!"

He shook his head in disbelief.

"Yeah, next Thursday. I propose to send you a contract if the rest of the board agrees, and I hope to God you do us proud. Don't mess with us!"

He stood up and offered me his hand. I shook it hard as I could. The others stood up too, and we all shook hands and said our goodbyes. Emily was still smiling. I gathered up my coat and briefcase and headed out with them, hugging Bonnie on the way.

Later that night, back in my motel room, I mulled over the events of the evening. I pulled back the curtains and watched the trucks shoot by in the darkness. The silhouettes of the trees shuddered, then stilled. The lights festooned around Bonnie's sparkled, and trucks lumbered in and out of the parking lot. I could hear faint strains of country music. It was so far removed from the skyscrapers of the Houston Medical Center, yet Professor Wilkinson's opinion had reached here. But they had not given in to him. Had I just imagined that? I tried to distract myself, but my mind was in turmoil.

There was a knock on my door. It was Ken Patel, the American owner of the motel. He was from Gujarat, a western state in India. He was shorter than me, plump, with a beatific smile.

"Hi, Dr. Mathur! I'm Ken Patel, remember me?"

"Of course! Come on in."

He stepped in and stood on the threshold.

"No, I got to go back to the front desk. Our front desk lady, she just didn't show up so I have to go back. But my wife, Sangeeta, she made these Indian sweets for you."

He produced a small tray of Indian sweets. They were bright yellow and white dumplings, decorated with slivered almonds and pistachios. I looked at them with astonishment.

"This is wonderful! I love these! Thank you so much!"

"You know today's Diwali?"

"Now I remember!"

"Yea, it's Diwali today. It's a holy day for us. You know, we make plans and start new businesses. It's a good day to start new projects."

Diwali is the Hindu New Year and celebrates the return of the great Lord Ram to his home of Ayodhya after fourteen years in exile. It's celebrated with fireworks, candles, lots of good food and prayers. I remembered the joyful Diwalis of my childhood, when my family sat and prayed together. I always sat next to Grandmother, listened to her recite, and savored the starchy fragrance of her sari.

"Yes, yes. I know."

"So how was the dinner?"

"Good! We had a good dinner, and I think I got along with them all."

"Then they will offer you the job. They are very honest, these people. If they say something, they mean it. Congratulations!"

"Thanks! I really hope it works out."

"How much time you got left on your visa?"

"Three months."

"No problem. But you should pray tonight. You know it is Diwali and you ate at the steakhouse. So you must pray and ask for forgiveness for eating meat. But I know you had to do it for your family. What a great opportunity! A new job on Diwali!"

I didn't know what to say.

Ken patted me on the hand and left.

"Remember to pray!"

After all the years in medical school, after the years in Bahrain, in London, in Houston, after the marriage and the children, after all the training and all the exams and interviews and licensing and paperwork, here I was, I thought, on Diwali day, in Hotspur, Texas.

Yes, I could make this work, but was I too quick to compromise? Quitting academics?

I suspected I *was* just a little bit dishonest, a bit of a charlatan. I had happily eaten meat on Diwali, *but,* I reasoned, *God already knew that.*

I turned out the lights and kneeled and gave thanks.

Thank you for this opportunity.

CHAPTER FOUR

Dr. Karl Becker

I disliked Karl Becker the moment I saw him. He was five inches taller than me, and four inches wider, a blond Hercules with curly hair and cool blue eyes that danced above a wicked smile that said *sucker*. I met him after my first weekend on call. He was in the hospital cafeteria, eating lunch with John Abbott, the administrator. He jumped out of his chair and lunged with outstretched hands.

"Karl Becker," he declared, shaking my hand energetically. "Sure'm glad to meet you! Welcome to Hotspur! Great job, this weekend! That boy just got out of ICU!"

"I know. I called."

"Man, you're just gonna *love* it here. It's *great* here!"

He squeezed hard. I squeezed back.

"Thanks! We're looking forward to it."

"Wife? Girlfriend? *Boyfriend?* Kids? All of the above?"

"What? Oh, yes. Got two girls, two and five years. Wife, wife's an architect."

"Two girls, eh? Gonna try for a boy?"

"We've got as much as we can handle."

"You look young enough. Plenty'a bullets left! Could *try!*"

"Maybe. Anyhow, I wanted to introduce myself."

"Know all about you. You're a gastroenterologist, internist, fixin' to do your boards and get certified. On a J1 visa, which means you need a waiver from Uncle Sam to get a green card and stay on in the great US of A. You want to hang around here for three years, get your green cards, then scram!"

"Well, that's kind of the idea but not so."

"Slam, bam, thank you ma'am!"

"No, no!"

42

"Hey, I just say it like it is. No BS, okay? You don't really care about this town and truth is they don't really care too much 'bout you. They need a doc, plain and simple, and you need a green card. You can come here, see a few folks, and then get back to Houston or Austin or Beverly Hills, hell, I don't give a rat's ass. Sit you down and have lunch with us! Hold on! You ain't *vegetarian?*"

He said all this so fast and with such a warm smile that I didn't know what to say or think. I shook my head numbly.

"Sit you down and git you some chicken-fried steak, looks like you need it. You scrawny! Your lady don't cook? Or don't she cook good?"

"No, no, just too busy finishing up my training. Missed too many meals."

Karl eased me into a chair, and with his hand on my shoulder, brought his face on level with mine.

"I'm gonna tell you something real important, now you're out of that damn training and in the real world. Listen up and listen good. *Never miss a meal for a patient!* You got that?"

I nodded, not at all convinced, but eager to avoid contradicting him.

"Never miss a meal for a patient," he repeated. "That's your lesson of the day! And I'll tell you more. Much more. Jus' keep listenin' and you'll learn plenty. Potatoes?"

"Thanks!"

I sat down and helped myself to chicken-fried steak and mashed potatoes.

"You follow sports? You know anything 'bout football? Guess not, bein' from India and England. Football is the state religion of Texas. Love it. Used to be the high school quarterback!"

I did not know, at that time, how impressive that was. So I lied.

"The *quarterback*. Whoa! So you were the big guy on the team!"

"You could say that. All the girls loved me. Had my pick an' I picked the best!"

He pulled back his sleeve and on his forearm was a heart with BETTY in it.

"Betty! She was the best! Cheerleader extraordinaire! Married her before I got into med school."

"So you were pretty young when you got married."

"You could say that. Had our first one a year later. Chad. Next one was Nate, and we got Nate in the middle of med school."

"How did you manage? Med school and two little kids?"

"Her parents. They would come and take Betty and the boys for weeks and I'd study. Studied my rear end off!"

"That's great," he continued, "having that kind of support. We had Jonah in Fort Worth after med school while I was in residency. Three boys!"

He put his fork down and reached for the meat. "Hope your girls don't look too much like you."

John Abbott stopped and stared at Karl. John was cherubic, blue-eyed, and sported a comb-over. He started to say something, then returned to his meal and kept glancing at Karl.

"What I mean is, you're not the best lookin' specimen. Face kinda like smushed brown paper. All Indians look like you?"

John Abbott half-opened his mouth but again said nothing, and resumed eating. I was piqued.

"Guess that's what Cecil Rhodes thought," Karl continued. "Made him feel superior. Made *all* the whites feel superior."

I looked around in astonishment. This was too much! John Abbott finally spoke up.

"You going to pass the steaks sometime this year?"

Karl helped himself first, then handed John the plate. John grunted.

"So who's this guy, Rhodes?" John asked, between gulps.

"Cecil Rhodes? Famous British dude, went to South Africa, *crushed* the locals, made them slaves, made *millions*."

I made an effort to move on.

"So you like it here, Karl?"

Karl smiled broadly.

"It's great. We love it. We bought us a great, big house up on Morgan Hill, thirty acres, wife and kids happy."

"What's it like to practice medicine here?"

Karl still smiled but looked away.

"I've got a great practice. Folks love me. You ain't a threat, no sir. Biggest problem's Doc Bulent. He's got a huge practice."

"I saw him walking in the hospital lobby. Didn't get a chance to talk to him."

"You saw that *gnome*? He's a damn *fraud*. Says he's a specialist. In oncology. Hell, he ain't even board damn certified in internal medicine, let 'lone any specialty. But he puts on all these airs and on his shingle says he trained in internal medicine and oncology. I wrote to his medical school and you know what? You know *what?*"

He stabbed a piece of meat and waved it at me.

"They said he never finished his training in oncology! So he ain't even board *eligible!* Puts up a damn shingle with ONCOLOGY written all over it, damn *liar.*"

"Well, that's wrong. That's false advertising. I read about that in the Jurisprudence exam."

"Yeah, everybody knows that. So I called the State Board on him."

"You called *the Board* on him?" I asked.

"Damn right I did. And you know what they did? Not a damn thing."

"Guess they gave him a warning or something."

"Shingle's still there. Didn't help any."

"Well, what about Dr. Kennedy?" I continued. "What's he like?"

"Ken Kennedy? He's a cripple. Got a real bad back, can't hardly get 'round. Sweats so hard you think he's run a marathon, but I think it's the narcotics, you know, the painkillers. He just sits in his clinic near the school and sees a few patients every day. Does what he has to do, then goes home, gets paid by the Charity Clinic."

"Do you think I can ask him for referrals? For GI stuff only, of course."

Dr. Becker guffawed.

"Kennedy's patients so piss-poor they can't even fill the medicines he writes for 'em. Hell no, they can't pay to see a specialist. But don't worry, you'll be jes fine here. You can see five or six patients every day and I'll see thirty or forty and I'll feed you a few consults."

I was stung and confused about what to say. I decided that it was too early to argue, and it would be best to humor him rather than confront him. Karl carried grudges; he had called the State Board of Medical Licensure on Dr. Bulent. Karl was very popular among the staff and the patients. His good looks and easy smile made him likable, but he was notoriously blunt. I made an effort to like him; after all, I was contracted to share the clinic with him.

"What you doing after lunch?" Karl asked.

"Going around the hospital."

"Wanna come see something? I got a little case. Want to see something *different?*"

"Sure."

45

The clinic was on the second floor of the hospital. His staff watched us politely, and he waved at them and sauntered into a patient room. There was a teenage boy and his mother in the room. They stood up immediately, the boy swaying, and his mother, half his height and twice his weight, stood stiffly. The boy wobbled and held on to the chair. He looked wary. Karl bumped fists with him but ignored the woman.

"Hey, this is my neighbor's son. His dad asked me to take care of his boy. Sandy, you ever done a fish hook?"

"Well, no. But I've read about them."

"Lemme show ya. It's Chad, right?"

"Chase."

"Yeah, Chase. Okay, Chase, just lie down on your belly. Dr. Sandy and me, we're gonna take that hook out, okay?"

The boy grunted and did as he was told. He was wearing an old vest and the fish hook had sunk into the back of his left shoulder. Around it the skin had swollen up and turned red. Karl gave it a gentle tug. Chase yelped in pain and tried to sit up. The woman held him down grimly.

"Okay, okay, just checking, don't worry. Hey, Sharon, I want iodine and lidocaine, gonna get this sucker numbed up."

The nurse nodded and selected a surgical tray.

"Yes sir, Dr. Becker. You want two percent or five percent lidocaine?"

"Gimme five percent," he said. "Stronger's better."

"With epinephrine or without?"

"Hell, I don't care. Give me what you got."

"Yes sir!"

Karl quickly scrubbed the area clean with iodine, ignoring the boy's whimpering.

"Big stick now!" he announced and before the boy could stiffen, he jabbed the shoulder and infiltrated lidocaine into the skin, raising a small wheal.

"The secret's to do it quick with the needle but slow with the lido-caine. Then once you get some lido in, you wait a few seconds then use the edges of that bubble to inject more lidocaine, so they only feel the first jab. So after that first jab you're always going in to skin that you already numbed up. Got it?"

I nodded. *I knew that.*

"With a fish hook, you gotta push the hook *in* then *up* to have it come out the skin again. Like so."

With a powerful twist, he pushed down on the stem of the hook and then up. The barbed tip of the hook popped right out of the skin about a quarter inch from the stem. The area was so well prepared that the boy didn't flinch.

"Now what you do is cut off the barbed end with a pliers, but before you *ever* do that do you know what you got to do first?"

"What?"

"You gotta get your eye goggles on 'cause the sharp barb can come off so fast it can get into your eye or face or somewhere."

We put on eye protection, and he snipped off the tip. It shot off and pinged against the cabinet.

"*See* what I mean?"

"Yeah, that was impressive."

"Nothing impressive 'bout that. Getting a fish hook out of the face or hand or finger, that's difficult. Got one outta woman's privates, now *that's* a story! This was easy."

He snapped off his gloves and threw them into the bucket.

"Give him the tetanus shot," ordered Karl.

"But his mother said he's up to date with all his shots!" Sharon protested.

"That's not his real mom, that's his stepmom. She doesn't know squat. Give him the tetanus shot. And don't bill for the visit, I ain't chargin' him."

"You sure?" Sharon asked. "He's got good insurance!"

Karl didn't bother to answer as he sailed out. He had a recklessly generous air that I envied. I wondered if I would ever be that confident. He went to his office to take a phone call. He was back in minutes.

"Hey, Sandy!"

"What?"

"Your wife just invited us to dinner with y'all, Saturday. We'll see ya!"

―――――――

Karl brought his family to our home that Saturday. He arrived right on time, at six in the evening, with his wife Betty, and sons Chad, Nate, and Jonah. They looked as if they had stepped out of a Norman Rockwell poster. Betty was as tall as Karl, blonde, blue-eyed, beautiful and warm, dressed in an elegant denim outfit. Their children were blonde, good-looking, and polite, and sat and smiled happily. Chad, the oldest, was fifteen and almost as tall as Karl. He was well built and had a blonde crew cut and an easy smile. Nate was twelve and wore glasses. He was much shorter and had shoulder-length hair and looked at everything with great curiosity. Jonah was ten, plump, and talkative. The boys wanted to see *Star Wars* so Priya and Anjali took them to the TV in our covered patio. The four of us sat down in the living room. Betty smiled warmly.

"How old are they again?" she asked.

"Five and two. Priya was born in London and Anjali in Houston."

"Priya is the older one, right?"

"Right. She was born at the Royal Cross Hospital in London, where I was working before we moved to Houston."

"So is she a British citizen?"

"No, it doesn't work like that. You have to live in England so long and pay taxes for so long, and there are lots of rules which means that basically you can't be a British citizen automatically even if you were born in England."

"What about the younger one? She was born in Houston, so is she a US citizen?"

"Oh, yes, she's a US citizen by birth. The United States is much better about that. She's an American citizen, no question about it."

"So why do you have to come to Hotspur and work to get green cards?" asked Betty. "Your daughter is a US citizen, so doesn't that make you all US citizens?"

It amused and irritated me that this great privilege was taken so lightly by those who grew up with it.

"She can sponsor us after she grows up, but not before she's eighteen or twenty-four, or something, I don't remember exactly how old. We didn't want to go back to India and wait twenty years."

"Well, we're sure glad to have you in Hotspur," said Betty, looking at Karl for support. Karl grunted and looked away and examined a coaster. Betty turned to Maya.

"So what are you going to *do* here? I mean, about your kids? There's no other Indian kids here."

"What if Priya and Anjali fall in love with a good ol' white boy?" Karl asked, slyly. "I got to ask. I got three boys!"

I was taken aback. It shocked me to think of my little girls as women

48

and then as women falling in love. I wanted to preserve them as they were.

"I don't know. I guess I would be okay with them marrying anyone, if they were good kids and if that was what they really wanted."

"You don't mind if they marry white boys?"

"No. So long as they're good kids, I really don't care."

Karl grunted. He thought of something else.

"So how'd the two of you get hitched up? Arranged wedding?"

I, too, changed gears. I had grown used to this question, but Karl was more abrupt than most.

"We were introduced by some family friends. We met a few times, dated, and then got engaged. We got married three months later."

"I thought you saw her for the first time when your daddy dragged her back from the bazaar and said, *here's you a wife!*"

"Now, *Karl!*"

"Just kidding, honey! Just kidding."

I laughed. Maya looked uncomfortable. I suddenly realized that she was not used to Karl's way of talking. I turned to her, shook my head and rolled my eyes, and she got the message. She relaxed a little and faced Karl with a brittle smile.

"It used to be something like that a long time ago," I said. "May still be like that in the villages. But in the cities, if you find someone yourself, that's fine, but if you *don't* find someone, then your family starts hunting for you. They ask around and try to find people you would be, you know, compatible with, and check with others to make sure that there was no scandal connected to the family, or criminality, or other bad stuff."

"Like what?" Karl asked.

"Well, mental illness, for instance. If there was a strong family history of severe depression or other mental problems, then the marriage might not get off the ground."

"Hell, I sure am glad they don't do that kind of thing here. I could never have gotten married!"

"You shush, Karl. You were never that bad!"

"What did your dad say when you told him?" he asked her.

"Nothing."

"Nothing!" Karl exclaimed with mock incredulity. "He said I didn't have a snowball's chance in hell of getting into med school and that you would be marrying a loser!"

"He never meant it!" Betty flushed hotly.

"Whatever. He was a sorry old such-an'-such, excuse my French. Couldn't get himself to give me a Christmas gift 'till third year of med school. What's your in-laws like, Sandy?"

"Oh, they're okay. We get along well. Her dad's an architect and her mom's an English teacher. In fact he was the chief architect of the city we grew up in, a place called Chandigarh. Her mom taught at a convent school run by Irish nuns."

"How old are they?" Betty asked.

"I'm not sure, but I would guess they're in their early seventies," I ventured.

"Mom did private tutoring from home for a few years after she retired a few years ago," Maya added. "She loved teaching English."

"Anyone else? What about your brothers and sisters, Maya?"

"One brother, he's a lawyer in India, and a sister. My sister works for a bank in Toronto."

"So I guess you don't really know anyone who lives in a trailer park, do you? Sandy's parents are both doctors, and you've got architects and lawyers. Damn!"

Maya looked at me, confused.

"What about you?" I asked. "I heard your brother lives in town."

"Yeah, Terry lives here now. Got him fixed up at First Bank of Hotspur, he's done well. Got a couple kids, younger'n ours."

Betty leaned in.

"Karl's the older of the two boys. We grew up together in Anson. His daddy was the Ag agent there."

"What is that?"

"The Ag agent is the, like, representative, of the Agricultural Department, of the government. Some kinda government deal."

"Part of the USDA," Karl explained. "US Department of Agriculture."

"Sure, I know the USDA. In fact, they're the ones who sponsored me to come here and work for the hospital. They're the ones helping me get my visa changed to a green card."

"Hell, if I'd known that I would've made sure you never came here!"

Maya and I froze, our mouths open.

"Karl!"

"I'm kidding, I'm kidding. You know that. I just say things."

"Karl likes to say things that shock people, y'all. Don't take him seriously; pay him no mind at all," Betty spoke hastily, sounding flustered.

I stepped in.

"I know Karl, I work with him every day. I know he kids a lot. It took me some time to get used to it. Is your office staff used to it?"

"Most of the time. Not all the time."

"Never a dull moment while you're around, eh, Karl?" I said, sarcastically.

"Told you, Betty!" Karl crowed. "He *loves* it! Well, tell us some more bout y'all. I want to hear more about how y'all got married. So your parents like, set y'all up and y'all got married, just like that? *Weird!*"

"No, it's not like that," I answered, uncomfortably. I shifted my chair closer to Maya. "We were introduced to each other by her first cousin, who worked in the same hospital as my mother. We met and went out together. I took her out for coffee, then for dinner, then another dinner. We had a good time together, liked each other, then we got engaged in Delhi. Three months later, we got married."

"You dated her before marrying her?"

"Sure. We don't have those arranged weddings anymore. If you can find someone to marry, then your parents will let you marry pretty much anyone you want to, but if you don't come up with a candidate by, say the age of twenty-five, then your family jumps in and starts hunting for . . . the right person."

"I don't think they wait till you're twenty-five," Maya added. "In my case they were talking about it after I turned twenty."

"You're so pretty you probably had 'em breaking down the front door, Maya! Now, Sandy here's an ugly mutt, what did he do to get someone like you?"

Maya laughed and shook her head.

"Karl!"

"Was his daddy rich? You was poor?"

"Well, no."

"Just wanted to get married? Change of scene? Don't give me the hooey about finding *true love.*"

"Well, Karl, I saw *ten* men before Sandy and he was the best of the bunch! He was gentle and kind, and I thought, well, I could *mould* him, you know."

Karl threw his head back and roared with laughter. Betty barely suppressed a chuckle.

"Mould him? *Mould* him? Like Jell-O in a mould! That's priceless!"

Karl turned to Maya, who had resumed her brittle smile.

"Hope you don't find my questions offensive. I just like to know folks."

"I don't mind at all," answered Maya, smiling tightly.

"So you were married in England?"

"No, Maya was in India and I came back, and we got married in India. In Delhi. We had a short but traditional wedding, just two days. The first day was the informal partying with a live band, and the second day there was a three-hour ceremony by a Brahmin priest in front of a fire and then a huge dinner."

Karl was not impressed.

"Hell, you sure couldn't a' dated her much or talked much then. Still think it's an arranged marriage."

"I don't think so," I argued.

"Well, that's all right. You know here in the US of A, with all the love and valentines and family values we have we still got a pretty high divorce rate. Know how much it is?"

"No."

"Fifty percent. *Fifty percent!* That means each wedding has an even chance of ending in divorce. That's pretty bad, if you ask me. Anyhow, that's life, don't get along, get someone else, just don't sit around and whine and mope, right Betty?"

"Karl's making fun of my parents, y'all," Betty said, shaking her head wearily and rolling her eyes. "My folks don't get along. Always yelling and fighting, neighbors calling the police on them. Worst-kept family secret of all time."

"No, the worst-kept secret was your brother," Karl chuckled. "Want to tell them 'bout him?"

Betty looked down and bit her lip and paused. She shook her head slowly, then looked squarely at Karl and said, "Karl, honey, maybe it's time for you to take a break."

Karl was about to say something but stopped. He sat at the edge of his chair for a minute, then stood up.

"Well, Betty maybe it is. Will you folks excuse me?"

Without warning, Karl reached for his hat. He put down his beer on a side table and used both hands to adjust his hat, a wide-brimmed weather-beaten white number with a brown band of sweat. I looked at Betty, puzzled. She was still sitting, looking down again.

"Karl sometimes likes to go and check on his patients in the hospital. Likes to surprise the nurses, just go down suddenly and just check on his patients."

Karl shrugged apologetically. "I just need a few minutes. Don't wait up on my account, go ahead and serve dinner, I'll be right back."

I was both surprised and impressed. In my conversations with Karl I had never sensed such a keen interest in his patients. *Never miss a meal for a patient*, I recalled. Yet, here he was, interrupting a meal for his patients.

It was a great idea, I thought, for him to go check on his patients. He had told me he avoided admitting patients to the hospital, so was he just being cautious? Something didn't feel right. Karl strode out. We heard his truck snarl to life and charge down the hill. Betty turned to Maya pleasantly.

"Honey, let's go lay the table and get the food going. Boys are hungry and Karl'll be right back."

Maya had already laid the table but got up and walked Betty into the dining room. Betty picked up some napkins and started placing one on each plate. Maya murmured thanks. I picked up my beer and followed them.

"How do you like the neighborhood? Made any friends so far?"

"Actually, yes. Sandy and I have met the Castleberrys and the Taylors, and the Templars have actually invited us for dinner next weekend."

"Tommy and Agatha *Templar*?"

"Yes."

"They used to kind of *own* this town. Really upper-crusty, old money, if you know what I mean. Own land and oil, had the insurance company, horses, you name it. Tommy sold the insurance business to the Castleberrys and is now retired."

"So you know them?"

"The Templars and Karl didn't hit it off right. Karl's a bit rough," Betty explained, "but he means well. You've just got to see that side of him. He sticks his neck out for others, really does. Cares a lot. Got a real big heart in there, he does, but tries to hide it."

"Sometimes he does a good job hiding it," I mumbled sarcastically.

Maya was appalled.

"Honey, I can't believe you just said that! What a nasty thing to say! If you've got something to say about him, say it when he's around, not behind his back."

My face stung, and I looked away. Betty smiled at Maya.

"Maya, Karl would hate it if I ever told you, but have you heard of the Citizen of the Year Award?"

"No."

"The Chamber of Commerce gives it every year. It's a big deal. I think Karl deserves to get it this year. You have to be nominated by a peer, someone in your own profession, so maybe Sandy could nominate him?"

I was taken aback. I wasn't quite sure what I thought of Karl, and I felt insecure drinking beer while he was caring for his patients. I made a show of arranging the plates as I wondered what to say. Betty moved closer to me.

"Sandy, I know he's rough on you, but have you heard about him and Herschel?"

"Is Herschel another doctor?"

"No, no. Not at all. Herschel was with Karl in high school when they were all growing up in Anson. Herschel was, ah, well, he was *African American.*"

She huddled closer, raised her eyebrows, and narrowed her eyes.

"He was *black*!" she whispered.

Maya and I looked at each other, surprised, not knowing how to respond. Maya recovered first.

"So Karl stuck his neck out for a black classmate?"

"Uh-huh. There was this, this black kid in his class. He was the state champion in the long jump or something like that, and he was good friends with Karl in high school, y'know, in his junior and senior years specially. Well, come close to graduation, turned out Herschel didn't have enough hours to graduate, so they told Herschel he wasn't going to graduate with the rest of them. Herschel told Karl, and Karl went to the principal. Karl was class president, of course."

"Of course," I said.

"So Karl went to the principal, and the principal says, 'Hey, I really want to help and all but Herschel has missed too much school on account of his state championship and training,' and so forth. So, guess what Karl says?"

"What? What did Karl say?" Maya was interested.

"'If Herschel doesn't get to graduate, then *none* of us will graduate. Not *one*. No one will attend the graduation ceremony.' *That* got their attention."

"So what happened?"

"Well, the school board met and went over things an' they decided that Herschel would have to take some makeup classes over the weekends and summer but he could get his certificate with the rest of the class."

"Bet Herschel was grateful for that," I said.

"Well, in those days we were kind of old-fashioned, you know, and schools had just been desegregated and all. We really didn't have a whole bunch of black kids in our county, but we all got along pretty well."

"So, did Herschel go to college?"

"Herschel never graduated. He was sure he wasn't going to graduate, didn't trust the school board I guess, and day before graduation, he got on a bus and skipped town. Never was seen again."

Betty looked back at our surprised faces with a shrug.

"Karl had to face the music, you know, sticking up for Herschel. Board threatened to expel him, but he's *like* that, he sticks by his friends. He doesn't care *what* color you are. He's a good guy. Hey, I should know, been married to him seventeen years," Betty said with a smile.

She held up her ring with a diamond the size of a bean. Her smile turned mischievous. Maya gulped.

"Don't *ask* how he could afford this, y'all, don't even *ask*. He worked day and night for it, moonlighting at nursing homes and ERs and such."

I avoided Maya's glare.

The children sallied back and forth into the sitting room, asking questions. They were boisterous and cheerful, and their lightheartedness was infectious.

"Mom, you should see their clothes!"

"They have the best little outfits!"

"Do you have *Aladdin*? The Disney *Aladdin*?"

"Where's Dad? Why isn't he here? Why did he go again to the hospital?" Jonah sighed.

"I'm hungry! When can we eat?" Chad asked.

"Why don't we serve the kids their dinner?" Maya suggested.

"Hey, great idea, if you don't mind serving twice," Betty said, "but we can all wait for Karl."

"Oh, I don't mind at all. In India, we routinely feed the kids first and the adults eat later. I do have some Indian food for the kids—not spicy at all—but I did get pizzas as a backup."

Betty and the boys were visibly relieved.

"Pizza sounds really good," they said together, beaming.

Karl returned about forty minutes later, flushed, swaggering, beaming, his good humor intact. I handed him another beer.

"Well, what is it tonight? Monkey brains for dinner?"

"Monkey brains! Why do you say that?"

"Ain't you seen Indiana Jones? *Temple of Doom*? Served monkey brains! Top-notch Indian cuisine for the Maharajas!"

"That was so over-the-top!" I said. "Most Indians are vegetarian, and others who eat meat don't even eat beef, and the Muslims don't eat pork. So in India we generally eat goat meat or lamb meat, at least where I grew up."

"No eyeballs in my soup, Maya, I'm allergic to them things! Give me croutons!"

Maya winced, then smiled.

"I'll strain the soup. Just for you, Karl."

"Attagirl, Maya! Well, I sure am hungry."

"Maya made chicken curry with rice, but no monkey brains. We had to buy local, and there were just no monkey brains."

"It was just a joke, Sandy. No offense."

"Sure. Let's eat!"

Maya had set an impressive table. She had a centerpiece with daisies, roses, and Angel's Breath. She had placed a cucumber and fennel seed salad at each setting. She had decorated her signature chicken curry with sprigs of cilantro and had made spicy cubed potatoes with sliced Serrano peppers. She had buttered flatbread and basmati rice, and it smelt as wonderful as it looked. Karl shook his head and held up his hands.

"Whoa! This is a feast! Maya, you have just gone overboard. You can't just sit down and eat something like this. We got to say a prayer first. Let's bow our heads."

We all bowed our heads.

"Heavenly Father, we thank you for your bounty and your love. We thank you for the land and the rain and the blessings you have showered upon us. Bless the Mathurs and bless this food that it might strengthen us to do thy duty. In Jesus's name, amen!"

"Amen!"

Maya liked the benediction and glowed after her cooking was praised. Long after dinner we sat at the table and traded stories about the children, about Houston and Fort Worth, and about the move to Hotspur. The Beckers told us about their wedding, his first practice in Frisco, a small town north of Dallas. Betty nodded approvingly.

"Yes sir, Karl's a good man, he really is," she announced, "and sometimes he can rub folks the wrong way, and then people get mad. But Karl's a *good* man!"

"Just have a habit of speaking the truth!" he interjected.

"You should help Sanju do that more often!" Maya said.

"Who is Sandroo?" Betty asked.

"Well, Sandy's name used to be Sanjay, and that is often shortened to Sanju."

"Why'd you change it?"

"My parents changed it when I was three or four because it had become too common. We had two other Sanjays in the family already."

"Well, I'm gonna stick with Sandy. Hey, do we get any dessert? I saved space just in case y'all believe in dessert like we do."

Maya had made rice pudding, decorated with coconut and slivered almonds. She brought it out proudly.

"You got any cake?" Karl asked.

"No, this is dessert. We don't have any cake. We do have some ice cream in the freezer, though."

"Forgot to tell you, I'm kinda lactose intolerant. Heck, gimme some, it looks so good. Red velvet cake's my favorite, for next time."

Karl said all this with a smile and regaled us with tales of how milk didn't agree with him. Before long, we were all laughing and Karl showed no signs of stopping.

"Lactose intolerant like you wouldn't believe! So much gas! Blasted the windows outta her folks' Suburban! They thought one of the dogs had been sick in it! Stunk up the place for days, an' I couldn't get off the dang WC. Had more gas than Oklahoma!"

"Karl, you gotta stop! These folks will never invite us all again!"

"They're gonna find out soon enough!"

"Anyone for coffee?" Maya interrupted.

Karl and Betty raised their hands. I stood up.

"How do you like your coffee?"

"Just like I like my women! *Hot and black!*"

I stood there, open-mouthed, while Karl roared. Betty shook her head. Karl mellowed after that. Later that evening he talked about himself.

"You got to forgive me," Karl said, leaning back and gazing at the ceiling. "Fact is, my daddy ran out on us when I was six. We had no money. Mother went to work and so did I. Worked every day at the Dixie Pig and the cotton gin, cleaned up, stacked stuff, washed up, waited tables. Kept studying, somehow. I reckon everyone calling me 'white trash' made me want so hard to be *something* it got me to medical school, just to stick it to them."

He swallowed and stared at me.

"Blamed myself for my dad running out on us. Maybe I still do. But that's another story."

I blinked and looked away. I was lost. I would never have told anyone that! Karl looked thoughtful and the room remained quiet. Maya broke the silence and spoke to Betty about the Hotspur Elementary School. Karl held up his cup for a refill. As I poured the coffee, I scrutinized Karl. So he had struggled for years. He had supported his mother and brother and pushed himself through medical school. He was crude but likable in a rough, disabling way. His sharp humor skewered everything and everyone, even himself. Reluctantly, I found myself being charmed.

He was honest *and* smart *and* funny.

Karl started talking again, and I glanced at Maya. She smiled broadly.

"That was too much information! Y'all didn't need t'know all that!"

Betty rose and set her coffee cup back on the table.

"I think we need to get going before Karl spills all the beans! We got a truckload of family secrets! We can save them for another day. Honey, are you ready to go home?"

Karl stood up and stretched.

"Yeah, I guess I am. Let's get the boys."

Betty offered to stay and help clean up, but we declined. We saw them off and returned. We talked about them as we loaded the dishwasher and wiped the table and countertops. Maya summed him up.

"He's crude and rude, and there's something weird about him, but I have to say, I like him."

I had wanted her to dislike Karl and validate my resentment, and I was disappointed. I had misjudged him. An awful realization hit me; there was more.

I was jealous of Karl.

CHAPTER FIVE

The Banana Splint Day

The next morning, I found Anjali sitting unhappily at the breakfast table. She pouted, her forehead creased, and her eyebrows rose toward her bangs as she hunched over her breakfast. She looked like a wilting button mushroom.

"What's up, Anjali?"

Anjali glared at her plate.

"Banana!"

Maya had placed a banana on her plate. Anjali detested bananas.

"Bananas are good!"

Anjali looked away.

"Try a few bites! You'll see! They're really pretty good!"

"No!"

I sat down and put an arm around her.

"Want me to peel it for you?"

She pulled loose.

"No!"

"You want some other fruit?"

"No!"

"What do you want to eat?"

"Waffle!"

I sighed. I knew that answer was coming. Anjali always ate waffles in the mornings, and Maya was trying to get her to eat more fruit. The banana sat alone on the plate, smiling insolently. Anjali pursed her lips and blinked hard, then crossed her arms.

"Okay, I'll go ask Mom if you can have something else. Just wait."

I found Maya getting Priya ready for school.

"She really needs to eat fruit. You know that. She eats waffles all the time and we've talked about it. Yesterday, she promised to eat a banana

59

for breakfast. So now she has to eat the banana first, then she can have whatever she wants afterward."

"Well, she's sitting there, pouting. You know what she's like, all angry and sad and silent. How about half a banana?"

"She should eat the banana. It's a small banana."

"She refuses. How about if I eat half and she eats half? Then she can eat something else?"

"No, she should eat the whole banana. She agreed to it yesterday. I want to hold her responsible."

"It's just a banana!"

"It's not *just* a banana! It's good, healthy breakfast food! And she should get used to it! And you should be supporting me, not helping her get away with it!"

I shrugged and returned. To my surprise, the banana was gone. Anjali sat there, smiling calmly.

"You ate it?" I asked, clearly surprised.

"Yes."

"Really?"

"Yes."

"Because you had promised Mom?"

"Yes."

I was impressed. Maybe Maya had a point. *Maybe I needed to be strict, like her, and get the job done. Yes,* I reasoned, *I needed to be stricter and raise the children lovingly, but firmly. Tough love, yes, that's the way.*

Visions of two obedient little ninjas appeared; they bowed deeply, and said, *thank you, venerable Father.* I was as easygoing as my parents, and I was hoping for validation.

"Waffle! With syrup!"

"What! You don't want another banana?"

"Waffle!"

"How about saying please?"

"Please! Waffle!"

I toasted her a waffle, still feeling the need to assert my superiority.

"How about jelly instead of syrup?"

"No!"

"Jelly tastes good! Try it?"

"No!"

I picked up the bottle and showed it to her.

"You like strawberry jelly!"

"No!"

"Okay, how about just a little jelly on the side?"

"No!"

"Some other jelly?" I asked hopefully.

"No!"

I reached for the syrup. Maya stuck her head around the corner.

"That's okay to give her syrup. But next time give her jelly."

I sat down with Anjali and we ate together. Anjali watched me wordlessly for most of the meal. I had a peanut butter-and-jelly sandwich and offered her a bite.

"No."

"You're very quiet today."

"I eating."

I watched her with amusement and imagined her developing jaw muscles contracting and relaxing. I admired her clay skin, clear eyes, and brown bangs.

"I born in Houston, right?"

"Yes, you were born in Houston."

"Houston, *Texas*, right?"

"Right."

"So I *Texan*, right?"

"Right."

She turned to look at me, puzzled.

"*So why I not blonde?*"

I smiled.

"I want blonde hair!"

"Maybe when you grow up."

Anjali returned to her waffle, unconvinced.

Maya walked in.

"Sanju, the ER called. You have a patient. Something about her hand."

"No problem. I was just finishing. I'll go brush and wash up."

I went to the bathroom and stopped short. In the wastepaper basket, sitting majestically on top of a mound of paper and plastic, was a banana. I snatched it up and went back to the dining room. I waved it under her face.

"You threw away your banana, didn't you?"

Anjali blinked but kept looking at me.

"No."

"Of course you did! What is this?"

She glared back at me.

"You just went and threw it away when I was talking to Mom!"

"No."

"You lied to me!"

"No."

I was exasperated. My daughter was challenging my authority. I had to do something drastic.

"Maya!"

No response.

"Maya!"

Anjali winced but stared back defiantly.

"Maya! Anjali threw away her banana!"

No response. A sneer started to form at the edges of Anjali's mouth. I knew that, inside, she was trembling. Or at least, I hoped she was. I gave her a stern look and waved the banana at her.

"You are in big trouble."

Maya appeared with Priya and sat her down.

"Priya, what will you have for breakfast?" Maya asked.

"Waffles."

"Okay."

"Maya, Anjali threw her banana in the trash!" I complained.

Maya straightened up and looked at Anjali, who promptly dropped her head and whimpered.

"Forget it. I'll deal with it. You've got that patient in the ER. Remember to bring that instrument to look at Anjali's ears, I think there's a hearing problem."

I was grateful to get away. At least in the ER, they followed orders. I grabbed my coat and left.

————————

"Hello, doctor. I'm Sam Rasmussen. This is my wife Bonnie. Thanks for coming to see her."

Sam was a tall, thin man with a goatee and a flop of untidy white hair. He held his hat in one hand and offered me the other. As I shook, I noted that his shirt said *Rasmussen Oilfield Supply*.

"How do you do? I'm Dr. Mathur. What's the problem?"

His wife stood up. She was a short, plump lady with a cheerful smile. She wore jeans and a button-down white shirt, and smelled pleasantly of mint.

"Doctor, I was gardening this morning, and I tripped on the patio and fell on my hand. Now it hurts and it's swollen."

I looked at her left hand. There were some abrasions on the side and deeper scratches on the forearm. The wrist joint was swollen and tender. I held her left hand gently and tried to move it up and down and side to side.

"I'm going to move your hand a little. This may be painful."

It was. There was very little passive movement possible.

"Let me check the movements of your fingers."

I held her wrist immobile and had her flex and extend the tips of her fingers. They had normal strength, but movement was painful. I checked her arterial pulses.

"When you bend or curl the fingers, that's called flexion, and you have two sets of flexing muscles, the deep flexors and the superficial set. The deep flexors bend the tips and the middle of the fingers and the others bend only the middle. So that's why I need you to first bend just the tips of the fingers then all the fingers together."

"Oh, I understand."

"And because you have good pulses, we know that your arteries are intact. They could get hurt or get cut by broken bones."

"Do I have broken bones?"

"I don't know yet. I told Ben, and he ordered the X-rays. Has Joe taken the X-rays?"

"Yes, about ten minutes ago."

"Then he should be bringing them back any minute now."

"We know Joe. Good man. Goes to our church."

Joe returned with the X-rays, fresh from the developing machine. He was a tall, lean man with white crew-cut hair. He had a lazy eye and moved his head in sudden bursts so I could never tell where he was looking. He used to draw blood samples without wearing gloves because, he said, he could palpate the veins better, and I had insisted he wear gloves, so we were enemies. Joe looked at me and said loudly, "Where's Doc Becker?"

I stepped forward and tried to take the wet films from him.

"I'm on call," I explained.

"Oh," he said, "Oh. Uh-oh. *Uh-oh!*"

He sounded extremely disappointed, but never actually said anything. He held on to the wet films and shook them one last time, then jammed them onto the viewing box. We all crowded around. I scrutinized the long bones of the forearm and the small bones of the hand. It was a sharp X-ray, well focused and centered. I found the fracture quickly.

"Tell us what's goin' on, Doc!"

"You have two long bones in the forearm, the radius and the ulna. The radius is the bone that goes from the elbow to the thumb side of the wrist and the ulna sits next to it and goes from the elbow to the little finger side of the wrist. The lower end of the radius looks like a triangle. Do you see it?"

They strained, then nodded.

"And there is a tiny crack in the triangle. Do you see it?"

"So I have a fracture?"

"Yes, you have a crack or a fracture in the lower part of the radius bone. It's called a Colles' fracture."

"Write it down, Doc. I got me a cousin is a vet, he'll be calling and he'll sure wanna know."

"Sure. The good news is that your fracture is undisplaced. That means that the bone pieces have not moved apart. The bone cracked, but the two sides didn't move apart. They're still in the right place. So all we have to do is put your wrist in a cast for a few weeks and it should heal right up!"

To my surprise, Sam clapped.

"Hey, that's great, isn't it, honcy?"

"But can I do gardening?"

"With your right hand,"

"But I'm left-handed!"

"Then it's going to be difficult. Maybe Sam can help you."

"Doc, I need to be her gopher?"

"Her gopher?"

"Y'know, like Sam go fer this and Sam go fer that and fetching stuff."

"I get it. You're her assistant."

"That sounds fancy. No, just gopher."

I reviewed her history. Bonnie was taking clonidine and a diuretic for hypertension. She was allergic to penicillin. She had a hysterectomy at age forty and bunion surgery at forty-five. Her physical exam revealed her blood pressure to be 170/90 millimeters of mercury.

"That's kinda high, Doc!"

"Yes, it is. Are you taking your medicine regularly?"

They exchanged glances.

"Well, that's been a problem. Y'see, she always feels so tired and sleepy."

"What he means is, when I take the medicine like I'm supposed to, I get sleepy and tired and can't hardly do nothing. All I want to do is lie down and sleep."

"And, boy, can she sleep!"

"Hush, Sam! So I take my medicine in the morning and then I try to take it again in the evening but I usually miss the afternoon dose. It's supposed to be taken three times a day."

"In fact, she gets so sleepy that she's always falling around in the house and the garden!"

"Well, how about changing your blood pressure medicine?"

"To what? It took us forever to get it right! Dr. Becker worked and worked at it. This was the best that we could come up with."

I hesitated. I realized that this was Karl's patient, and I didn't want to intrude.

"Well, how about you discuss it with him when you see him for a follow-up visit? After all, you'll be seeing him about removing the cast."

"Yes, that's a good idea. We'll talk to him," Sam said.

I set about applying the cast. I rechecked the X-ray and confirmed that the bone fragment was not displaced. I took three rolls of Plaster of Paris bandages and soaked them in a bucket of water for five minutes. I had Ben hold her left hand with his right hand as if he were shaking hands with her and had him apply gentle traction. I had Sam grip her elbow and hold it steady. I quickly unrolled a sheet of cotton and wrapped it around her forearm and over her wrist. I tore off smaller strips to encircle the base of her thumb and up an inch. I fished out the Plaster of Paris rolls and squeezed out the extra water and unpeeled the edge. I applied the bandages in a tight spiral, starting just below the elbow and ending by looping around the base of the thumb. I applied more Plaster of Paris bandages to overlap the first one, all the while smoothening out the surface with warm water. The end product was a glossy white cylinder that started in the upper forearm below the elbow, tapered at the wrist, ended in mid-palm, and included the base of the thumb. The thumb stuck out at an angle. I made sure that she could wiggle the thumb and the fingers.

"How's that?"

"Feels warm!"

"Yes, it's supposed to feel warm. The Plaster of Paris gives off heat when it gets wet and as it sets. Keep your forearm elevated. The forearm is the part from the elbow down to the hand."

"How long do I have to keep the cast?"

"Four weeks. Then you can come and see Dr. Becker, and he can decide whether the cast should come off or not."

I slipped my fingertip underneath the shell. The fit was snug but not too tight.

"We need it to be snug but not *too* snug," I explained. "If it gets too tight, it can cut off the circulation and the muscles and skin can shrink badly. That's a serious complication. So if it starts hurting or feeling too tight, call me right away. Or just come back here, and we'll take care of it."

Ben cleared away the bucket, the water spills, and the discarded packaging. I finished the paperwork and wrote out a prescription.

"This is a prescription for Tylenol with codeine. It should help with the pain."

"Is that dope?"

"Dope? You mean, a narcotic?"

"Yes, dope?"

"Well, codeine is similar to morphine and, yes, it is a narcotic."

"Then I don't want it," Bonnie responded. "All those things make me loopy. I've got ibuprofen and such at home, I can take that."

"As you wish," I said with a shrug and tore up my prescription, feeling a little humbled.

"Dr. Becker is comin' to see her afore she goes," Ben informed me. "He just called from home, asked if you could please wait. Just wants to say hi to the Rasmussens. Says he was comin' here anyway."

I didn't like that. *He was coming to check on me, my work, and to make sure I hadn't taken his patient.*

"Sure," I said. "Of course."

I pretended to be busy with paperwork but found it galling. I had taken care of things and resented Karl coming down to approve of everything. I bit my lip and decided not to say anything sarcastic. Soon, Karl burst through the door and high-fived Ben. Swiftly, he hugged Bonnie and shook Sam warmly, grasping his forearm. He turned and patted me on the shoulder.

"Hey, buddy! Just thought ah would say *Hi* to these folks! Hope you don't *mine?*"

I was convinced Karl was manipulating his accent, like a master politician. Reluctantly, though, I admired his performance. *Medicine is the art of keeping the patient amused while nature performs the cure*, Voltaire said. I settled back and watched. Karl pulled up a stool and hunched over the cast. He had Ben focus the lamp. He rotated it around gingerly and twisted his head around. He ran his fingers over it and then inserted his small finger in deeply like a dipstick at one end then the other. He grunted approvingly.

"Yep, good space. Good cast! Where's the X-rays?"

"Joe took 'em back to send to the radiologist in Abilene."

"Well, get 'em back in here. I wanna look at them!"

Joe appeared promptly at the door with the X-rays. He had a grim smile.

"Here's the X-rays, doc. I don't know, I'm just a tech," Joe said, his eyes dancing, "but I kinda think there's *a second* fracture that you *missed, Dr.* Mathur."

I was stunned. My mouth went dry. I opened and closed it. I felt everyone watching me. To my horror, Karl looked at the X-ray and nodded. Joe scrambled to point out his finding and consolidate his victory. He pointed with the tip of his pen to the lower end of the other long bone, the ulna. There was a fine white line at the base.

"There's a fracture of the lower end of the *ulna* as well, and I reckon it's displaced."

Karl looked at the X-ray sternly, then shook his head. Joe moved in for the kill. He stood next to Karl, nodding ingratiatingly. His bony finger jabbed the spot on the film and pointed out the faint white line. Karl stepped back and said nothing. I froze. I could see the Rasmussens looking at the cast suspiciously.

Joe hissed.

"He *missed* the ulnar fracture! There it is, broad as daylight! See it?

Says he's a specialist, but misses a fracture! *Misses a fracture!*"

Karl shrugged.

"Sure is a tiny fracture. But sure as heck ain't displaced. It's okay."

"Do you think Dr. Mathur needs to *remove* the cast?" Joe asked eagerly.

Karl looked unperturbed.

"Hell, no! Great cast! Couldn't put a better one myself. And that tiny podunk fracture? Heck, *anyone* coulda missed that tiny crack!"

Joe recoiled in disappointment. Karl struck again.

"*I* coulda missed that tiny ulnar fracture! Yep, even *I* coulda easily missed it! The Colles' fracture is the one that counts, treatment's the same. Interestin' findin' sure, but hell, makes no difference to the treatment. Makes no difference! That there is a mighty fine cast!"

Joe gathered up the X-rays, crestfallen.

"I'll send these off to Abilene."

"I don't care. Whatever."

Joe threw me disdainful glances as he withdrew, like a hyena denied its prize. *You missed the second fracture*, I sensed him to say, but I didn't care. Karl had tossed him aside, and was reading my notes and praising my cast. He did not bother to thank Joe.

"*Damn* good positioning an' cast. Good job! Specially for a damn specialist!" he announced, his voice booming out into the hospital.

He tossed the clipboard to Ben, wiped his hands on his trousers, and whipped out his sunglasses. He turned, and winked at me before he slipped them on and strode out.

I could have hugged him.

———

I went upstairs to the clinic and sat in the back of the office and gulped coffee. The back of the office was screened from the check-in window by three cupboards and offered some privacy. The area was about ten feet by ten feet and included Heather's workstation and two sagging chairs. A coffee machine was perched next to a small sink; cardboard boxes served as side tables. Old files and defunct desktop computers, fax machines, and keyboards were piled against a wall. Heather had discovered a manual in a cupboard and returned slowly to her desk, appearing engrossed in *The International Classification of Diseases, Version Five*. She ran her finger down the index and doggedly ignored Karl, who glared at her as he sat in his favorite corner, near her chair, and kicked it petulantly. Heather looked up and spoke to him.

"Dr. Becker, I found your disease! You have Infantile Behavior Syndrome!"

Karl stopped kicking her chair and turned to me.

I was still berating myself for missing the second fracture. I knew that it was small and that it didn't change the management, but it bothered me a lot. *I should spend more time reading X-rays,* I thought. *Maybe I had been in a hurry to give them a diagnosis and show them how smart I was. Maybe I need to review my whole book of orthopedics.*

"Sandy, let it go!"

I looked up to see Karl towering over me. He held out a donut.

"Have a donut."

"No, I don't want a donut. Thanks, though."

"Don't be such a tight-ass. Have a donut."

"No, I don't want a donut."

"You're still beating yourself up about that fracture, ain'tcha?"

"I guess."

"Course you are. We all do. We always want to be right, all the time. Hey, we're doctors."

"I don't understand how I missed that fracture."

"You're just human. You can get it wrong. Happens."

"What if I miss another fracture? What if I miss something else?"

"You're human. You're going to miss stuff."

I scowled.

"Better get used to the feeling. You're going to screw up sometimes, just like the rest of us. Doctors ain't perfect."

"I should have been more careful."

Karl shrugged.

"Have a donut."

I reached up and accepted it. It was remarkably good. A wave of cinnamon and sugar woke me up.

"That's really good!"

"Krispy Kreme donuts. Got 'em from Brownwood."

"I've got to get Maya to try them."

"That's my philosophy. When you get your ass whupped, get a donut. Know why? Cause that way, at least one end's happy."

━━━━━━

I checked Anjali's ears that night. One side was pink and normal and the other was red. I looked again to make sure I hadn't missed anything. I was still smarting from my embarrassment. Anjali had to go to bed early, without any TV, as punishment for throwing away the banana and lying to me. Anjali curled up, turned to the wall, and whimpered. I drew the curtains, turned out the lights, and tucked her in. I sat on the floor, my back resting on the side of her headboard. I imagined her chewing her lips and blinking back tears, determined not to cry. I understood how she felt.

"Mom gave me banana. For lunch," she complained.

"I know."

"I made a painting. For Mom!"

"I know."

"She gave me *banana! And no TV!*"

"I kind of slipped on a banana today."

She paused.

"You not lookin popperly?"

"I guess I wasn't."

"You hurt?"

"A little."

"I didint cwy. You don cwy."

"I'm proud of you. Sometimes things don't work out, and we just have to deal with it. You had your banana and I had a fracture. We both made mistakes."

I waited. Silence.

"And our mistakes were caught."

I remembered my anguish, and wondered if Anjali had felt something similar. I thought of something.

"Hey, do you think we can call it our banana splint day?"

She was already asleep.

CHAPTER SIX

Everything but Money

Francisca Sophia de Allende was the receptionist in the administration section of the hospital, but everyone thought she *was* the administration. Her fine looks, graceful demeanor, and family connections ensured that nothing went through her department without her approval. She smiled as I entered and waved toward the silent air conditioner.

"We've no air-conditioning, sorry. Budget cuts, doctor. We're trying to save money and can't afford to have it repaired."

She shrugged dramatically, sending ripples through her silk blouse.

"Mr. Abbott is expecting you. Some more bad news, I expect. If it wasn't for bad news, there wouldn't be any news at all!"

I sat down on a mousy brown sofa and kept sinking. I grabbed the armrest.

"Can I get you something to drink? Coffee? Water?"

"No, no, I'm fine," I mumbled as I pulled myself back up.

"He won't be long. I think he's on the phone with the lawyer. You know, the one who's doing your immigration work. Boy, is he expensive! He bills us by the hour and his bills show up every couple weeks!"

I didn't know what to say.

"I bet you're here because they're having trouble paying you, am I right?"

I concealed my surprise, then admitted, "Yes, and I don't know what to do."

She nodded knowingly and looked away. As I waited, I studied her.

Francisca Sophia was in her mid-forties, I guessed. She was slim, attractive, and possessed trophy hair. It was chestnut brown, impressively straight, and shiny. Several locks curled across her forehead. A lot of her time was spent tossing that hair around elegantly, scooping it up behind her with both hands, and coaxing it into a ponytail. Minutes later, she would release her hair, angling her head sideways and snapping it like a whip. When it found its way to the front of her blouse, she watched it indulgently until it had inched back too far, then tossed her head, throwing it back majestically, crushing the insurrection, exclaiming, "Hah!"

Her other preoccupation was the state of her skin.

"My *God*, Dr. Mathur, *look* at the *state* of my *skin*," she complained loudly, displaying a vast expanse of limb and shoulder indulgently.

I pretended not to gape. Her skin shone like satin. Francisca Sophia dug into her purse and retrieved a small urn of buttery white myrrh. She lifted the lid. The room became fragrant. Giving it her fullest concentration, she rotated a finger and teased a wave off the surface. She inspected it for flaws, eyebrows arched, lips pinched, torso taut, breath held. Keeping the finger under inspection, she replaced the myrrh in a box and slid it into a recess in her purse, still remaining wondrously poised, with a pearl hovering untouched at the tip of that finger.

It was at that moment that the phone rang.

She didn't flinch. She ignored it.

The telephone rang and rang. Francisca Sophia blew gently on the dewdrop.

The phone rang some more then stopped, then rang again. It was ignored. Francisca Sophia examined the pearl minutely.

The phone stopped ringing.

The fax chirped, and a few pages flopped onto the floor. They stayed there. Francisca Sophia proceeded to rub the mousse into her left hand. First the back, then the front, then the spaces between her fingers and finally, climactically, on her fingers, ending with a searching examination of her nails. A man appeared at the window with a form. She flexed and straightened her fingers. She blew on her fingers as she played them in the air like a piano.

The phone rang again. After a few rings, she scooped it up, and waved at the man at the window who waved back.

"Hotspur County Medical Center, where we are *dedicated* to your *complete* health, *good morning*, how may I help you?"

She covered the mouthpiece and winked.

"I kill them with my kindness!"

Everyone loved her.

John Abbott, the administrator, ushered me in. John was a genial man with an impish smile. We shook warmly. His office had thick shag carpet in mousy brown and wall-to-wall wood paneling. A small window looked out behind him onto an abandoned approach to the hospital and was almost hidden behind striped chocolate drapes. An air conditioner sat beneath the window and spluttered. The roof was low, and John warned me about hitting my head against the ceiling fan that sported four small light bulbs. They provided all the light in the room. John's desk had a telephone and a lamp with a green shade but no bulb. Certificates from the Rotary Club, the Jaycees, and Lions International hung at odd angles in between hunting trophies.

"Hey, Doc! Just got off the phone with your immigration lawyer! He says everything's going ahead smoothly!"

"Great! Thanks for pushing this through," I said, and sat down at his desk.

"Sure! Doc, we're going to get this done for you! You don't worry about a thing!"

I coughed and cleared my throat.

"I wanted to talk to you about my salary."

"Your salary?"

"Yes, my *guaranteed* salary. In my contract, I was guaranteed seven thousand a month, but I haven't been paid for three months. I'm still borrowing from my dad!"

John bit his lip and nodded.

"Yeah. Well, you see, Doc, it's like this. We got everything but money! We got patients, we got staff, great nurses, great doctors, we got a first-class lab and patient rooms! But, problem is, we're in a financial hole. We're deeply in debt and we just don't have much money."

He looked me in the eye and threw up his hands. I shook my head.

"How can that be? I mean, you have staff and doctors and ambulances and all. How do you pay them?"

"We pay hospital staff with loans from the bank. Yes, we collect taxes from everyone who lives in the county. We're a tax-supported hospital. But we have also taken out a bunch of loans, and we're just barely making it!"

I took it in slowly. John went on.

"The doctors make money by seeing patients and billing their insurances. The insurance companies pay the doctors directly. We don't make money on outpatients, we make money on inpatients. We charge the doctors a small rental fee for the clinic space, three hundred a month. That's nothing. So they don't depend on us."

"But I do."

"Yes, because you're new and you don't have many patients. Hey, it takes time to build a practice."

"So how will I get paid until I start seeing enough patients?"

"Well, that's what we're here for! We said we were going to support you and by golly we are!"

He looked earnestly at me.

"I begged Tommy Cooper at the bank for one last loan to pay for your immigration lawyer. *Fifteen thousand!* Way I see it, that's critical. No green card, no Dr. Mathur! We're betting on you big time. That's where the money is going, to your lawyer, instead of you."

John went on.

"Your lawyer charges fifty bucks an hour! Says he's one of the few lawyers in the country that knows how to do this visa deal! Sends me a bill every week! Tell you the truth, Doc, I had no idea it would cost this much!"

"So how will you pay me?"

"Your lawyer is costing way more than we figured. So we've less in the kitty to pay you."

"How much less?"

John scrunched up his face and looked up for a moment. Then he looked at me.

"How about two thou a month, Doc?"

"Two thousand a month less or two thousand a month total?"

"Two thousand a month total. But just for now. As soon as things get better, we will start paying you everything."

I looked at him. I could not think of anything to say. I needed the visa converted, and I needed to pay my own bills.

"Bill, I made seventeen hundred a month as a doctor in training! I can't make two thousand a month as a full doctor!"

"Don't worry about it, Doc! You're going to be just fine! Everybody likes you! It's just a matter of time. Your clinic practice will get you the big bucks!"

He looked at my face and went on.

"Hey, don't feel so bad. You got a great job, a great family, great place to work! Everything but money! Look, I can help you get a loan from the bank if you want."

"No. No loan."

"Okay, fine. Look, your house rent is five hundred, right?"

"How do you know?"

"Hey, Doc, this is a small town. Everyone knows everything here. Okay, so five hundred's the rent. School's free, food's cheap. Keep your expenses low for a while."

I looked at him.

"You can do it. You got immigrant grit."

I managed a grin.

"Doc, let us work on your green card first. You gotta have that to stay in the US of A. We'll keep working on your pay."

I thought about how I would break the news to Maya.

"Bill, I appreciate all you have done for me and I appreciate all the hospital is doing for me. Tell me, *why* is the money situation so bad?"

John slumped. It was his turn to remain silent.

"The bottom line, Doc, is this. You know all the patients in the hospital? You see all those inpatients? Well, most of them's Dr. Bulent's patients. Dr. Becker has a few patients too, but really almost all are Dr. Bulent's. Problem is, we haven't billed for Dr. Bulent's inpatients in *three years!*"

"What do you mean?"

"Dr. Bulent admitted lots of them and discharged all of them, but he never did write any discharge summaries on any of them! So we can't bill Medicare. Not until Dr. Bulent does all the discharge summaries for the *last three years!*"

I began to understand. I knew that a hospital couldn't bill Medicare until it had a discharge summary and discharge diagnoses, but I had never heard of not billing for three whole years! Medicare was the colossus amongst insurance companies nationwide, and in Hotspur not billing Medicare meant not collecting a dime. *For three years!* It was astounding!

"Oh, now I understand. You have to have the final diagnosis for every case before you can bill their insurance."

"Yeah. Almost everyone here in Hotspur is on Medicare. Either that or Medicaid or nothing. You know about DRGs?"

"Not really."

"DRGs are Diagnosis Related Groups. Medicare and all insurance pays you depending on the final diagnosis. You admit someone for a urinary infection, you get paid so much, whether you keep them in a day or a week or a month. Doesn't matter how long and what you do. You can give them a real high-powered high-dollar antibiotic or you can give 'em penicillin, doesn't matter. You get paid the same. Because it was the same diagnosis, same DRG, same payment."

"So what about for a myocardial . . . heart attack?"

"You get paid more for a heart attack, of course, than for a urinary infection. But again, you can give 'em the highest priced clot-buster in the world or you can give an aspirin, it doesn't matter. Paid the same for a heart attack whether you did a lot or did diddly-squat."

"So the final diagnosis decides what the hospital gets paid."

"That's it."

"So how has the hospital survived? No billing done for three years?"

"We're living off taxes and loans. Loans from the banks in town, donations from wealthy families, and from cutting down our staff and paying everyone less. No Christmas bonus for four years!"

"Why don't you lean on Dr. Bulent to just finish his paperwork? Maybe even threaten him with suspension?"

John laughed.

"We tried it. You don't know ole Doc Bulent. He just stormed out and discharged everyone and didn't admit anyone for a couple weeks. Our census was zero. We surrendered."

"Can you take legal action?"

"His daughter's a lawyer and she keeps sending us these legal notices. We can't afford a lawyer to scare him! I bite my tongue and keep calling him politely, reminding him."

"What does he say?"

"Says he's too busy. When he even returns my calls."

John stood up and turned and looked out the window.

"I know it looks pretty bad. When I came here a year ago they said this place was about to fold. I've kept it going. I got faith. I got faith in God, and my Christian brothers and sisters. I got faith things will get better."

I stood up.

"I got faith in you too, Doc. I got faith in all our docs. But sometimes I think we need a little help from the boss man above."

John turned to look at me and sighed.

"Truth is, we're in deep trouble. I hate to say it, but we are so tight, so tight, we may not make it."

"What do you mean? Close the hospital?"

He grimaced.

"We've got to do everything to keep it going. The town *needs* this hospital. We have to do something drastic!"

"Drastic? Like what?"

"Board's going to ask to *raise the property tax rate* to fund the hospital. People gonna *hate* it, that's going to be *ugly!*"

He grinned sardonically.

"In case you haven't noticed, people hate paying taxes, so they'll likely reject the tax hike. I don't know how we're going to get out of this mess."

A thought struck me.

"Well. I don't have that much work these days. How about if *I* went to medical records and read Dr. Bulent's charts and dictated the discharge summaries? You think that would help him? He's so busy seeing patients. And I don't need to be paid anything extra, I would just do it for the hospital."

John looked interested. He nodded his head slowly.

"Well, that's a thought. Why don't I put it to Dr. Bulent and ask him? I'll let you know what he says."

"Will Medicare pay for patients from three years ago?"

"Yes, they will!"

"Then tell Dr. Bulent I could start today."

After the meeting, I went up to the clinic. It was a Tuesday morning, and there was a relaxed atmosphere. Dr. Becker held court. He sat in his corner in the back of the office and rested his feet on a box. Heather looked relieved to see me. Kendra was getting coffee. Karl had *Guns And Ammo* open on his lap and waved his mug at me.

"Hey, Sandy! My man!"

"Hey Karl!"

"How the hell are you, Sandy? How's your family?"

"Doing well. Still getting unpacked. Takes more time than we expected."

Karl was sitting near the coffee machine, hunched over the local paper.

"So how was the meeting?"

"What? You mean, with John Abbott?"

"Of course. What other meeting, Einstein?"

I paused, then decided that honesty was the simplest option.

"Yeah, I met John. We talked about finances."

"So did he offer you two thousand or two and a half?"

I gagged, and stared at him.

"That's okay, you don't have to answer that in front of everyone. Should have figured you'd be touchy about money."

I poured myself some coffee. Karl addressed Heather and Kendra. Kendra paused uncomfortably.

"Hey, you know what I was thinking? I was thinking, why does Sandy spend so much time in the clinic and the hospital? Why don't you go home for lunch with the missus and the kids, Sandy?"

"I do go home sometimes."

"You eat lunch here a lot! Why do you stay here so much? Free food? Come on! Don't you like your wife?"

"Of course I do!"

Heather turned around.

"Dr. Becker, what a thing to say!"

"I don't remember asking your opinion, Miss Heather Nosy Watson!"

Heather stiffened but stood her ground.

"I was just asking Sandy—*Dr. Mather*—why he didn't go home to have lunch with his wife and kids. He doesn't have any patients here!"

"Well, I want to be available if they show up. I want to be here so they can see me if they want to."

Heather jumped in.

"And he wants to be here so you don't butt in and see them before he can, Dr. Becker!"

Dr. Becker glared at her but said nothing. Heather turned back.

"Forget it. So all's well with you and the missus?"

"Of course."

"It's a small town. People notice things."

"I'm fine! We're fine! You're right, I should go home for lunch. I guess I'm insecure."

Karl grunted and looked away.

"I guess it takes time to build a practice."

"Sure does! Took me two years! Old man Bulent fought me tooth and nail!"

"Over patients? Surely patients are free to go where they please?"

"Dr. Bulent grabs them so tight they fart!"

"Dr. Becker!" Heather said.

"What? Like no one ever said any cuss words here before? Before Dr. Royal College Mather showed up?"

Heather scowled.

"Personal physician to the holy Queen, is he? We can't cuss anymore? Give me a break!"

Heather rolled her eyes and turned back. Karl laughed.

"Hey, did you guys like my Sea-Doos?"

"Well, water scooters and jet skis are fine but no waterskiing for me," I said.

"Great! Well, Betty'n me, we're setting up another weekend for the whole office at Scarborough Lake. We plan to have us a fish fry and get out the water scooters and all our toys. You all come!"

"Thanks a lot!"

"Yo, Kendra! My patient showed up yet?"

"Yes, sir. Room Two."

Karl lumbered up and took a long draught of coffee. He wiped his lips with his hand.

"Duty calls! Got to go save lives!"

"Dr. Mathur, Maya is on line one."

"Thanks."

I took it in my office with the door closed. I knew what she was going to ask.

"So how was your meeting with Mr. Abbott?"

"Oh, it was interesting. I learnt something about the hospital and its finances. They're in deep trouble. They haven't billed Medicare for most of their inpatients for *three years!*"

"That's crazy! Why not?"

"Most of the inpatients are Dr. Bulent's patients and he hasn't written any discharge summaries in three years!"

"So that's why they're in such a bad shape! They're in trouble, everyone knows that."

"I found out."

"So what about your guaranteed salary?"

"They are spending a lot of money on the immigration lawyer and so they're really tight."

"So how much *will* they pay you?"

"Two thousand."

"*What!* You got seventeen hundred in training!"

"That's what I told him. He just said there's no money and we really need green cards right now more than the money."

"So how long will this go on?"

"Don't know. But I offered to help them get the discharge summaries done so they can get paid."

Maya remained silent.

"Are you on call this weekend?"

"No."

"We need to take Anjali to see an ear specialist. I'm worried about her hearing."

"I checked her ears. One's slightly inflamed, the other's fine."

"I'm worried. Can you set up an appointment? I want you to come."

"Of course. The one they recommend is a Dr. Argyle in Abilene. He may be hard to get into this week, but I'll get an early appointment."

"I can't believe they can only afford to pay you two thousand a month. But for how long?"

"Like I said, he didn't say."

"Until they pay the lawyer?"

"I suppose. We definitely need that completed. I can't move anywhere else. If the hospital collapses, I'll need to find another place that will sponsor me for a green card."

"That won't be easy."

"It will be very, very difficult. Also, this hospital has been very prompt in getting the lawyer hired and starting the process. I really think they mean well."

"I can't believe that they haven't billed for Dr. Bulent's inpatients for *three years!*"

"It's a big blow for a small hospital like this. It could end it for them."

"So what do we do?"

"I don't know. Wait it out for now. At least get the green cards, even if there's no money."

"John Abbott seems to be honest. I like him. You know, I can tell about people. I feel we can trust him."

Maya had met John when we had come to Hotspur to find a house.

"I like John, too. I feel he's trying to help us. *Everything but money,* he said."

Maya sighed.

"Did you get the milk?"

"Sorry. I forgot."

"Well, that's okay. We need sugar and cereal as well. The girls want Lucky Charms."

That evening we sat on the porch and watched the sunset. We sipped hot tea and watched the shadows lengthen over the brush and the retreating wind tickle and tease the mesquites. We wondered how we would manage on two thousand dollars, and I dreaded the thought of calling my father again. Maya drained her cup and smiled.

"I'm making chicken spaghetti tonight. Can you bring some Italian breadcrumbs? The girls really like breadcrumbs in their pasta."

"Sure. I'm going to write a list so I don't forget anything."

"Don't forget the list!" Maya teased. I grinned.

She stood up. She was beautiful. She had smooth tan skin, short dark hair, a sharp nose, and perfect teeth. She had been my copilot through a lot of turbulence and kept me calm and motivated. She had maintained her attitude and her figure, and was proud of both. Many neighbors had reminded me how fortunate I was. When I had suddenly proposed to her in Delhi, in a taxi as we snaked through traffic on our way to dinner, I had braced myself for waves of uncertainty, but none had come, and I remembered that. *I was always comfortable with her.* We had good times and bad times; moving from London to Houston had been very stressful, but we had been optimistic. Foolhardy and optimistic. *You grow up in India,* I thought, *and you better have contacts or optimism. We can tough it out here, we can make it work. I don't want to give up and go back. Indians seem to do well in America, and in every country except their own.*

I went to the girls' room. They had bathed earlier. Priya was sitting in bed, reading, and Anjali sat in the corner by the big window, surrounded by dolls. There was a soft glow in the room, and their faces gleamed. The room was warm and moist. I inhaled and waited for them to notice me. I was in no hurry. The smell of shampoo and talcum powder was always pleasant.

Minutes later we were huddled in Anjali's corner while Priya explained with relish how Maya had unplugged the toilet that morning and then how they had spilled glitter glue all over their carpet. Priya gurgled with excitement and Anjali nodded vehemently and looked at Priya and then at me, to make sure I understood. She said nothing but contorted with glee and clapped. Priya became serious.

"Mom's always doing projects with us!"

"I know! I wish I could, too."

"Why don't you?"

"I've been getting back late. I get tired and sleepy. But I will, I will."

Priya looked at me, disbelievingly.

"Really?"

I winced.

"You should come back early."

"Yes, but sometimes people get sick at the wrong time. Just as I'm ready to go home, they show up!"

"Can't someone else do it?"

"There's only one doctor on call after five, so if someone shows up late then the doctor on call for that day has to stay back."

"What about the others?"

"They go home and rest."

Priya pondered this.

"So what if you're the one on call and you're tired?"

"You try to rest whenever you can."

"But what if you're in the hospital and you have to see sick patients and you're tired?"

"I drink coffee. Lots of coffee!"

"So coffee makes you strong?"

"Well, it wakes you up a little. Makes you less tired."

"If you're tired, you should tell them you have to go home to sleep!"

I smiled.

"Sometimes you can, sometimes you can't."

Anjali spoke, her brow furrowed, jabbing at me.

"Sleep! You sleep!"

"We can all get some sleep after dinner. But first we have to go to the Shopping Basket. Want to come?"

"Yes! I've got money!" Priya cried.

She opened her Lisa Frank bag and pulled out a purse. She fished out a dollar and waved it.

"Look! A dollar!"

"What are you going to buy?"

"I don't know. Something! Something I can share with Anjali."

"Okay. And maybe I can start the goodnight story in the car."

I strapped them in the back seats. Anjali had a car seat and Priya had a booster. I reversed out of the driveway with elaborate slowness. I was sure the neighbors were watching. I've always been a slow driver. In India, there was so much traffic that there was no option but to drive slowly, and in America, I was cautious because I had seen too many catastrophic wrecks.

"Mom is *much* faster!"

"Mom is too fast!"

"Mom can drive and sing!"

"I'm going to tell you that story. Do you remember the beginning of the Akbar and Birbal stories? Who was Akbar?"

"The king of India!"

"Yes, he was the most famous emperor of India. Who was Birbal?"

"His best friend!"

"Yes. He was Akbar's best friend but he was also Akbar's prime minister. He was the one who gave advice to Emperor Akbar."

I remembered my grandmother telling me these stories at night when I was a little boy. She used to sit at the end of the bed in the darkness, her clear voice repeating the opening phrases. I loved repeating it; it always reminded me of her, and it was a family tradition.

"Many years ago, in the times of the Mughals, there was one emperor of India who was the best, and his name was Akbar, and he was Muslim. His prime minister was Birbal, and he was Hindu."

"Tell us the one where he fell into poo!"

"You already know that one. And it wasn't poo!"

"Tell us that one! Again!"

Priya waved a small fist and egged Anjali to nod in support. I knew there was no escape. I would have to tell the poo story. I drove past our neighbors and down the hill on Cottonwood Avenue to Commercial, and made a left past Steiner's Automotive and Mitsy's Beauty Salon. People waved to me and I waved back.

"Who was the greatest emperor of India?"

"Akbar!"

"Who was his prime minister?"

"Birbal!"

"Correct. And one day the famous King Akbar decided to make fun of his friend Birbal. So in front of everyone in the court, Akbar said, 'you know what, Birbal, last night I had a dream.'"

"He was dreaming of poo!"

They doubled up in anticipation, their eyes glittering, waiting for the word.

"Akbar told Birbal in front of everyone, 'You know, Birbal, I had a dream. We were walking together and there was a pool of clean perfumed water and there was another pool of dirty stinky water.'"

"No! No! Not dirty water! It was poo!"

"Okay, one pool had nice, perfumed water and the other one had poo!"

The girls rocked with laughter.

"It was full of poo! Full of poo!"

"Yes," I said, resignedly, "it was full of poo. In fact, it was full of stinky green poo!"

"Eee-yoo!"

"With bubbles!"

"Did the poo go up to his face?"

"Yes! Into his nose!"

"No!"

"Into his eyes!"

They suddenly became serious.

"But then what happened?"

"Akbar said, 'I dreamt that I fell in the pool of clean water and you fell in the poo!' Everyone in the court laughed at Birbal. Then Birbal said, 'Excellency, I too had the same dream. I, too, dreamt that we were walking together, and there were two pools in front of us.'"

I pulled into the parking lot, parked, and continued.

"Birbal said, 'I also dreamt that you fell in the clean water and I fell in the poo. Then we got out, and you licked me and I licked you!'"

They clapped and hooted with delight.

After we walked into the store, I left the girls in the magazine and stationery section, next to the customer service desk. The clerk was always friendly and promised to keep an eye on them. I had not made a list but remembered the Lucky Charms, the milk, and the sugar. I found them and returned.

"Whoa, organic milk! Man, that's expensive!" the checkout clerk said. "You sure you don't want regular? Hospital don't got money!"

I stared at her in surprise. She was a plump teenager, with glasses and pierced eyebrows. Her dark hair was in braids and fell over her bare shoulders. She kept looking straight in front and I wondered whether she was really talking to me.

"You want me to go get you regular? You get a gallon for $2.99."

"No, this is fine."

Priya came up.

"Can we buy some stickers?"

"Nope."

"Can we have some ice cream?"

"Nope."

They looked up coyly and swayed slightly.

I stood firm.

They sighed audibly and swayed a little more.

"Can we have the stickers if I pay for them with my dollar?"

I was tired. I relented.

"Well. I've paid for the milk and cereal and sugar. Go ahead and pay. We have someone waiting behind me."

Priya strode up to the cashier and handed over the stickers and the dollar. The cashier rang it up.

"Dollar eight," she said, sounding bored. She looked straight ahead and held out her hand at a right angle.

"*What!* It said 99 cents!" Priya objected.

"Tax."

Priya turned to me and asked, "What's *tax*?"

I started to explain, but the cashier broke in.

"You want it or not? There's other folks waiting."

The cashier looked in front again. There was a couple behind us.

"No!" Priya burst out in a fit of pique. "I *don't* want it! It's not *fair!* It's not fair to put *tax!*"

There was a chuckle behind me.

"Well, *she's* Republican!"

The couple standing behind us introduced themselves. The lady was short, had unkempt white hair, and wore a T-shirt that said WORLD'S BEST GRANDMA. Her husband was at least a foot and a half taller; he wobbled from side to side and had a walker. He had bright blue eyes, a two-day stubble, and wore overalls. They were in no hurry. They talked to us as the cashier rang them up.

"Name's Johnson, Dave Johnson. This here's my wife, Mamie. You must be the new doctor. Well, welcome to Hotspur. We sure hope you like it here."

"I have liked it so far."

"How's your practice building up?"

"Slowly."

"Well, I may be coming to see you. Got a problem with my legs. Anyhow, you best get on home, those little girls look mighty upset!"

Priya was still fuming when we reached home.

"Tax! That's *not fair!*"

———————————

Maya had an urgent message for me: call John Abbott.

"Hey, Doc!" John couldn't contain himself. "You'll never believe what just happened! I told Dr. Bulent what you said and he went berserk! *Berserk!* Didn't want anyone looking at his charts! Screamed at me and threatened to quit the hospital and said he would slap us a lawsuit so big it would make our heads swim!"

"What did you say?"

"I told him, 'Doc Bulent, go ahead, we already hired a lawyer.' He said, 'You're kidding.' So I said, 'I will personally fax you the legal retainer receipt.' He said, 'You're bluffing,' so I faxed it over."

"Did he realize it was for my immigration lawyer?"

"Nope! Five minutes later he calls back all sugar and sweetness, reckon he called his lawyer daughter in California, and changed his tune. He's in the building *right now,* in Medical Records!"

"Right now? In the evening? In Medical Records!"

"You betcha! He just called, complaining there's poor lighting and no pens, no paper, no nothing! Heck, he ain't ever used it in three years is why there's nothing there!"

I pictured Dr. Bulent scribbling away furiously in a dismal corner of Medical Records.

"We can start billing tomorrow! There's no time limit on Medicare billing! There's a three-month limit on Medicaid, but the heck with that! *We can start billing Medicare tomorrow!*"

"That's great, John! Then maybe you can pay me!"

"You and everyone else!"

John hung up. I turned to Maya .

"Let's increase Priya's allowance. Two dollars."

CHAPTER SEVEN

Bait and Hook

My increasing availability led to a gratifying improvement in my practice: the numbers increased slowly. I sensed discomfort in the office when one of Dr. Becker's patients came to see me, but when one of Dr. Bulent's patients made an appointment, there was jubilation.

"Hey, you did it, Sandy!" bellowed Karl, giving me a high-five. "Goddamn it, you got one of Bulent's patients to come to you. Took me *months* to get my first Bulent patient."

We were in the office by Heather's desk. Karl scraped mud off his boot with a tongue blade and tossed it into the bin next to Heather. She jerked, turned to complain, but said nothing.

"Thanks," I said.

"He won't like it, you know. Just be prepared."

"Prepared for what?"

He shook his head and looked away.

"Just be prepared."

The new patient was David Johnson, whom I had met at the grocery store with my daughters. He was the former chief of police. Mr. Johnson was over six feet tall, brawny, bald, and rough-hewn. Canopies of skin covered his eyes, and dunes and craters decorated his forehead and nose where skin cancers had been cut out. He nodded and held out a big, fleshy hand.

"*Pleased* t'meet you, Doctor!" he announced. "David D. Johnson. Call me DD. And this here's Mrs. Mamie Johnson."

Mamie was barely five feet. She had white curly hair and wore cats-eye glasses. She wore a Hotspur Hornets shirt and a picture badge of her grandson holding a baseball bat. She was heavy on the hips and rocked back and forth, like a bowling pin. She gave me a firm and knotty handshake.

Osteoarthritis of the hands, with nodules.

"Pleased to meet you too. Thank you for coming, Mrs. Johnson. We met at the Shopping Basket."

"Some doctors don't like to have patients bring their wives," Mr. Johnson said.

"Oh, I don't mind at all. I think it's good to have an extra pair of eyes and ears in the room."

"Well, how about that, Mama? I like this little guy already! Doc, I need you to fix my feet. They're hurtin' me all the dang time. Ole Doc Bulent tried and tried but he jes couldn't fix it. Said he was goin' to send me to Scott and White Clinic in Temple, but I said, 'Whoa there, there's this new guy in town. Lemme see if he's got any good ideas 'bout fixin' this.' Feet been burnin' up for weeks and weeks."

Mr. Johnson had a history of poorly controlled diabetes. After a general exam, I sat him up, put on gloves, and peeled off his socks. The room suddenly smelt like a dead rat. I steadied myself and examined his feet carefully. His toes were deformed and overlapped. I pulled them apart and saw rivulets of thick gray pus in-between and underneath the toes like two *W*s. The undersurfaces of the toes and the ball of the foot had ulcerated. The skin had peeled away and the maroon dermis was exposed, with beads of blood where the socks had stuck. Mr. Johnson remained silent, but his cherubic wife kept up a good-natured patter.

"Sorry 'bout th' smell, Doc!"

"No problem."

"Doc, I been telling him to put Camphor-phenique on them things! He's jes stubborn as a mule, he is! No wonder they stink. Won't change his socks, neither."

"Yes, I do change 'em, Mother," DD said.

"Ever' Sunday mornin' before church!"

"Anyhow," I interjected, "right now they're definitely infected. Being diabetic, your feet are prone to getting infected. You have to keep them dry. So no socks, just wear open sandals or flip-flops, and clean your feet with soap and water and then with peroxide. Then you need to put some anti-fungal ointment in between your toes."

"What kind of soap, Doc?" Mamie asked.

"Oh, any kind. It doesn't matter."

"Well, I want to do zactly as you say to do, Doc. Lever soap be okay?" Mamie persisted.

"Yes, that'll be fine. Use Lever soap."

"*Any* kind of Lever soap?" DD asked.

"I would 'ave used Dove," said Mrs. Johnson with a sniff, "with moisture."

I looked at her. She was unconvinced. My credibility was on the line.

"Lever soap," I stated firmly, "without moisturizer."

She gazed back sadly, shaking her head.

"What about the anti-fungal deal, Doc?" DD asked.

"You can buy an ointment for athlete's foot from the pharmacy or grocery for about seven dollars. That will be cheaper than my prescription. Let me write the name of the non-prescription one for you. The fungal infection opens up the skin and then bacteria infect it, so the first thing to do is to get rid of the yeast. It loves to grow in the moist spaces between your toes, so keep them dry. Use a hair dryer if you can. I also want you to take Cephalexin five hundred milligrams four times a day for ten days. I'll have my nurse call it in for you. Which pharmacy do you use?"

"Bob Haseltine's."

"We'll call it in."

"Is it real high?" Mamie asked.

"No, it's a generic. Not expensive. I always try to write generics."

"Good deal, Doc!" DD said, relieved.

"See you back in two weeks."

———

The letter came soon after. It was in a stiff white envelope. The name NADINE BULENT, JD, A LAW PRACTICE was imprinted in the upper right corner. Heather handed it to me wordlessly in her office. Karl chortled and peered over my shoulder as I opened it. I scanned it quickly.

Dr. Mathur,

It has come to my attention that you have been seeing patients of my father. This is illegal and must stop immediately or we shall be forced to initiate legal proceedings against you. We are prepared to forgive you this once as you are new to the area, but if this happens again, you will be served formal legal notice.

We will inform the Texas Medical Association of your unprofessional conduct. They may investigate you and your medical license may be withdrawn. Your career depends upon your choices, and we will not hesitate to prosecute you to the fullest extent of the law.

Yours,
Nadine Bulent

I looked up, astounded.

"They're not his patients! He doesn't own them! They're not cattle!"

"Tell him that!"

"I will!"

"Won't do any good," Karl said. "He's jus' an old dog that keeps barkin' all the time. Says *he* will see his patients all the time, in clinic or ER. He's crazy."

"I thought we scared him with the immigration lawyer," I said.

"His daughter saw through it in two clicks. Bulent's still doing his records, though."

"What's this about reporting me to the State Board?"

"Routine stuff. She reports you to the State Board, they investigate you. They call the patient, patient says they wanted you, they drop the matter."

"So what's the point?"

"Oh, you know, you throw enough shit, some might stick. If they investigate you they might find something else! Might find out you're a child molester after all."

He grinned. He was enjoying this. I shook my head.

"Remember, he's working on his records. Been working hard as a one-legged man in an ass-kicking contest! Doesn't want *you* to look at them. You got him there, buddy. Forget it."

But I seethed. How could he do that? Was it ethical? What if one of his patients came to the ER? Could he really always be on call for his patients? And here he was, threatening me with legal action just because of a patient I saw? Reporting me to the *State Board* and threatening my license? What if they investigated me and found something minor and held up our green cards? My head pounded with the injustice of it all.

Karl slapped me on the shoulder and sat down.

"Get over it, Sandy. Docs are like that. We get territorial. It happens."

"It's wrong!"

Karl shrugged.

"Sometimes doctors are like regular folks. They don't like other doctors poaching. Docs are competitive."

I shook my head. *This was arrogance.*

"You just ain't been a doctor long enough."

———————

I spoke to Maya later. We were cleaning up after dinner. She shrugged.

"Forget it. Worry about your family first. I'm more worried about Anjali."

"But what if he starts some legal action?"

"Let him. You haven't done anything wrong, have you?"

"No! But how dare he threaten me! I have never said anything to him, and his patient came of his own will to see me!"

"Sometimes you hide the truth or you tell little lies. Tell me now, did you provoke him?"

"No!" I answered vehemently.

"Then don't worry about it. Go and get the girls to brush their teeth. Get them to bed!"

That night they asked for another Akbar and Birbal story. We were in their bedroom, the lights off, the waning sounds of public radio lingering in the air. Moonlight gilded the room, snaked up the bedposts, and spilled onto their wall art. The girls stirred and rolled with a palpable reluctance to admit the day was over and kept checking to see if I was still there, sitting on the floor by the door, sullenly inhaling the last of their soap and shampoo. I was still angry about the letter, and revised it again in my mind.

"Are you still there, Dad?" Priya asked.

"Yes."

"Are you going to tell us a story?"

"Yes."

"I wan Akba Beeba story," Anjali declared.

"Which one?"

"That one when Akbar gets angry with Birbal and tells him to go away," Priya said.

"But you've heard it so many times!"

"We love it!" they protested.

The moon vanished behind a cloud and plunged the room into total darkness. I waited for my eyes to adapt and tried to clear my mind. *How dare he be so arrogant?* Priya coughed theatrically and I forgot about Dr. Bulent. I started with my usual preamble.

"So who was Akbar?" I asked afterwards.

"He was the king of India!" Priya said. Anjali nodded.

"Yes, he was the emperor. An emperor is a very big king. He was the greatest emperor of India. And who was Birbal?"

"Birbal his, his best friend!" Anjali said.

"Well, actually, Birbal was his prime minister. That means that Birbal was his best friend and closest advisor. Birbal was the man who gave him advice on things."

"About what?" Priya asked.

"About how to run the country and about how to run his life and everything."

"When you tell *story?*" Anjali asked, peevishly.

I cleared my throat.

"Many, many years ago there lived in India a great emperor called Akbar, and his . . ."

"His best friend *and* prime minister, Birbal!" Priya announced, reconciling accounts.

"Yes, exactly. Birbal was a very wise man and gave Akbar good advice about everything and usually Akbar listened to Birbal, but not always. One day, Akbar found this poor, dirty beggar wandering through his palace. The beggar had a big, ugly beard and was wearing torn, dirty clothes and smelling bad, and Akbar got very angry."

"And told him to get out!" the girls sang out.

"And the beggar said, so where should I go?"

"The beggar was actually Birbal!" Priya told Anjali, conspiratorially.

"I know," Anjali nodded, sagely.

"And Akbar said, go stay in some shelter or guesthouse or dormitory or some such place. Somewhere where you can stay for a while and then go on your way. And the beggar—"

"Who was *Birbal!*" they said, happily

"Yes, who was actually Birbal, said, 'Well, your grandfather lived in this palace, and then your father, and they came and lived here and left. So they all came and stayed for a while and then left. They were guests, not owners. So this palace is actually a hotel, a shelter, not a palace. So we all are the same, we come for a while and we stay and then we leave. We are all the same, we live in shelters, and we are all travelers.'"

"Trav-lers," echoed Anjali, sleepily.

"Then Akbar understood that Birbal wanted him to be kind and to share and not be proud. Birbal wanted Akbar not to be selfish and wanted him to share the nice things he had."

"In the Akbar and Birbal stories, did Akbar ever get angry with Birbal?" Priya asked.

"Many times."

"But he always forgave him?" Priya questioned.

"Yes. Akbar knew that Birbal was saying and doing the right thing. So he would sometimes get angry but he would always understand later."

"So if we do the right thing and say the right thing, then the king will always like us, even if he doesn't like us right away?" Priya wondered.

"I guess so. You know, there's a message there for me, too."

"Goodnight, Dad," Priya yawned.

"Goodnight, pumpkin."

I turned to Anjali's bed. She wasn't moving. I kissed her forehead and went to Priya. She threw her hands around my neck as I kissed her.

"I *love* your stories, Dad."

The phone rang around two in the morning.

"Dr. Mathur?"

"Yes?"

"This is Clint in the ER. Are you on call?"

"Yes."

"We've got a young kid in here. Got a fish hook stuck. In his *ear*."

"In his ear? A fish hook?"

"Yep."

"He was fishing at two a.m. and got a fish hook stuck in his ear?" I asked.

"Wail, he was done fishin sundown. Bin trying t'get the thing out by hisself. It's not pretty."

I sat up. I remembered Karl's instructions. Fish hooks are like question marks, with barbs pointing backward from the sharp ends, to snag tissue and prevent removal. I shuddered at the thought of someone trying to wrench it out of his ear.

"Any bleeding?" I asked,

"Whole ear's a bloody mess!"

"He's not Dr. Bulent's patient?" I inquired hopefully.

"Nope. Already checked."

"I'll be right there."

I dressed silently and crept into the kitchen. I checked on the girls. Maya called out.

"Are you going to the hospital?"

"Yes," I whispered.

She sighed.

"Drive carefully. Lock the door."

I let myself out through the back door, locked it, slid into my Toyota, and drove down the hill. The neighborhood slipped away, serene and silent in the moonlight. In minutes, I pulled up in the hospital's parking lot. I was surprised to find three trucks there, with people milling around. They wore jeans and vests and cowboy hats. There was a strong smell of fish and beer.

"Hey, Doc! Thanks fo' comin' in!"

"Yeah, man! 'Preciate it!"

"Kevin's a-waitin for you!"

I nodded to them and hurried inside the ER. There were even more people inside. The examination room smelt of brackish water and rubbing alcohol. In the center, his head hung low, was a thin teenager, a mop of waxy blond hair covering his face. He tilted his head and covered his left ear with a wet mold of toilet paper, mottled brown and red. He looked up as I entered, then quickly looked down again.

"Hey, Doc! This here's Kevin Cisneros!"

The boy looked up and shot him an angry look.

"My name's McKenzie! Kevin McKenzie!"

A woman detached herself from the others and waddled forward. She was short and buxom and wore frayed shorts, a tank top, and a baseball cap that said DIXIE PIG DINER. She chewed gum as she spoke.

"Doctor, this here's mah son, Kevin. Ah used t'be McKenzie, but now I'm Cisneros. Kevin's bin adopted bah mah husband, so he's Cisneros."

"I'm McKenzie, Mom! I don't want to be Cisneros! You can be Cisneros if you want, but not me!"

A man stepped forward. He was over six feet, in jeans and sleeveless vest, with a muddy white cowboy hat. He smiled as he offered his hand.

"Sam Cisneros, Doc, pleased t'meet you. Ah'm his dad, or least, ah think so. Ah'm legal guardian, since his daddy ain't nowhere t'be found."

"That ain't true!" Kevin protested weakly, still looking down.

Clint, the nurse, stepped forward. He was a wiry man with a halo of curly grey hair, grey eyes, and a perpetual grin. He wore sunglasses backward on his head at all times. He handed me a form on a clipboard.

"Doc, Kevin is fifteen so we need his parents to sign for whatever you want to do. Here, I'll put the big light on the boy."

I scanned the form. Kevin was indeed fifteen years old. He lived on Nueces Street, did not take any prescription medicines, had no known drug allergies, and had never had any surgeries. He had been fishing on Scarborough Lake when he had tried to fling out a fishing line and had hooked his own left ear. He had tried to pull the hook out but it was too deep. The ear had ballooned and bled profusely. His mother had tried as well, but had only made the bleeding worse and the ear tripled in size and throbbed with pain. They detoured home to find some ice and pack the ear before coming to the ER.

"He wus trying t'show off t'his girlfren'!" his mother explained.

"No, I wasn't!"

"Yes, you were! Lissen t'your mother!"

I introduced myself. I had Kevin lie down on the gurney, face down, and asked everyone to leave except his mother. She hovered over to his right side and I approached his left ear. A mass of toilet paper was still clamped over it. It was wet from the ice and bloodstained. I lifted the soggy mass. He cried out, turned, and covered his ear with his hand. He glared at me.

"*Shit!* It *hurts!*"

"It's okay, sunshine! Doc knows it hurts! He's going to be ever so careful, right, Doc?" his mother said.

"Right, Kevin. I really need to take a good look at that ear. Just put down your hand and let me look."

Kevin glanced at me and then looked at his mother. After hesitating, he removed his hand and settled down. I soaked the paper with sterile saline and peeled it off. The mutilated ear came into view. I had prepared myself and did not blink.

"*Sweet Jesus, Kevin!*"

His mother covered her mouth with her hand. The left ear was grotesquely swollen and reddish purple. The hook was stuck in the pinna, the soft fleshy part of the ear that hangs down. The hook had entered through the back, and the tip was buried inside the swollen mass. The bloated ear was distorted shut, and a shiny two-inch wooden painted fish with bright red stripes and bulbous eyes hung down, exactly like a large earring, trailing six inches of fishing wire.

"That's the bait," his mother explained proudly. "Kevin made it hisself!"

I stepped back. It looked like a fish was leaping out his ear. I was half appalled and half amused.

"Well, I'm just going to do a brief exam and then I'm going to clean it up and take out the hook."

"Is it going to hurt?" Kevin asked.

"A little. I'm going to inject some medicine to numb it up first, then I'll work on it."

"I don't want it to hurt!" Kevin cried.

"Calm down, Kevin. Ah know this doctor an' he's good. *Real* good. An' he's gonna to take real good care of you. He ain't gonna to let you hurt."

I had never met her before, and it was a fair bet that she had never known of my existence until that hour, but I accepted the compliment and smiled.

"Kevin, just stay as you are. I'm just going to listen to your heart and lungs from the sides and back," I explained, showing him my stethoscope. He settled down. I turned to Clint. "Clint, I'll need a small suture tray with two percent lidocaine and no epinephrine. Make sure there is no epi in the lidocaine. And I'll need a really small scalpel blade, something like a two or three millimeter blade."

"You want your magnifyin' glasses?" Clint asked.

"Yes," I responded, "and I'll need you to come to the head of the table and hold the boy's head."

Kevin jerked upright, alarmed.

"I ain't doin it, Maw! I ain't doin' it!"

His mother stared at him for a few seconds, exasperated. She suddenly lunged forward and slammed him down with the flat of her hand. His head was jammed down on the pillow, and his skin creased under his mother's fingers.

"*Ow!*"

"Now, shut up!"

Kevin was silent thereafter, mumbling and sobbing softly, but was otherwise fully compliant. I sat down on the stool and trained the light on his ear. Clint took over from the mother and gripped Kevin's head firmly, anticipating trouble. I cleaned the ear and the adjacent part of the face and temple with alcohol, then with iodine, then with alcohol again, erasing the stain of the iodine. I used a very small needle, twenty-five gauge, to inject lidocaine at the base of the ear, taking care to infiltrate slowly. Kevin yelped, but Clint was prepared. The boy's mother half rose, then settled back down. I injected the lidocaine under the skin in front of the opening of the ear, where the ear attaches to the face, because that's where the major nerves lie. For good measure, I also injected in a clockwise manner all around the base of the ear. Soon, the only sound was Kevin's breathing and sniffing. I lifted Kevin's ear carefully.

No response.

I tweaked it a little.

Still no response.

"Okay, it's numb. Give me the scalpel."

I turned the earlobe over and palpated. I pulled on the stem of the hook and could feel the tip of the hook tenting. I made a tiny incision, starting at the point of entry of the hook and going toward the tip. Kevin remained silent. I pulled again. The hook stayed in place. Clint peered.

"There's lots of blood clot in there, Doc! Guess you got to go deep!"

I nodded and sunk the blade a little deeper and tried again.

"Doc, go for it!" his mother urged, wearily. "It's three in the morning, an' ah gotta get t'work in Brownwood at six!"

I cut deeper and deeper. I felt sure I would come out the other end. Where was the tip? Had it broken off? Had the family done something foolish? Was it lying free somewhere in the hematoma? I suddenly felt metal. I flung down my scalpel and pulled on the stem. Gradually, majestically, the tip came into view, rivulets of blood running down the tented tissues. I pulled it some more, and pushed back on the tissue, so that the hook and the barb were clearly above the surface. Clint handed me a pair of fine-tipped pliers, and we both put on eye protectors. With my left hand, I reached forward and snapped off the tip. With a *crack*, it shot up and hit my goggles. His mother hadn't missed a thing.

"Good thing you had them glasses on, Doc! Else you'd be headin t'Abilene wi' a fish hook in yer eye!" she said.

I pulled the metal stem out easily.

"He needs a tetanus shot. I'm going to write him some antibiotics. Have him come and see me in three or four days for follow-up."

The family trickled back in. Sam Cisneros came up to me and grasped my shoulder.

"Thanks fo'helpin him, Doc!"

"You're welcome."

"Hate t'git you outta your house this early."

He hesitated.

"Ah ain't got much money, Doc! Can't pay you, lease not this month."

Kevin looked up and muttered.

"Or this lifetime!"

Sam winced.

"Ah know the hospitals tight, ah know they ain't payin you. That hook, ah tried maself, ah jest cannat git that hook out of ma boy."

I shrugged.

"Sam, I'm a parent too."

"Ah pay you, promise, pay you later. Doc, ah jes don't have much! Too many bills awready."

"Sam, don't worry."

He scrutinized my face, then admitted.

"Kevin's acshully Doc Bulent's patient. But ah awready owe Doc Bulent a bunch. Figgered we try you."

I stared at him. I was shocked and angry. I glared at Clint, who shrugged helplessly. I spoke coldly.

"You should have told us the truth. We would have called Dr. Bulent."

Sam shook his head.

"Sorry, Doc. Ah owes *him* a bunch."

His face brightened.

"We're all going to switch *t'you!*"

"Dr. Bulent might not like that."

"We ain't cattle. He don't own us. We wanna to come t'you!"

I was too tired to argue. I started writing in Kevin's file. I documented his juvenile status and the permission from his parents, noted his history and examination. I checked his vaccination record. Clint got Kevin ready for discharge. I imagined the next legal letter from Nadine Bulent.

"Doc, don't be scared of Doc Bulent!"

I looked up, surprised. Sam swaggered as he adjusted his hat.

"He ain't the *king* of this place. We ain't *beggars*."

Sam warmed to the subject.

"He came from California, mebbe he go back to California! All these big docs *come and go!*"

I nodded and returned to my paperwork. I wrote details of the wound and the procedure for removal of the hook. Kevin's mother spoke up.

"Can't stay here forever, Doc."

I looked at her thoughtfully and nodded.

"That's very true," I said softly.

She coughed impatiently.

"No, I mean, I gotta get t'Brownwood by six. Hurry up th' damn paperwork."

CHAPTER EIGHT

This Is Spinal Tap

The next night on call was worse. I was called in at one o'clock in the morning. I trudged through the parking lot, avoiding the family members, and labored up the ramp to the sliding doors. Karl was there. I stopped, surprised and confused. He saw me and sprang up from a stool in the corner. He scowled, his face flushed, eyes bloodshot. His hands trembled; he whipped them behind his back and snapped.

"You didn't have to come in for this!"

"But I'm on call!"

"Yeah, but you're a *specialist*. You don't know how to deal with kids."

"I can assess them and if they need to be transferred, I can ship them!"

Karl threw his head back in disgust.

"Ship them! You think we're a hick hospital in a hick town, so whatever. We just *ship everyone*, right?"

I kept my voice calm.

"If it's too complicated for us to handle, we *should* ship them where they can get whatever care they need."

Karl glared at me and shook his head. His eyes widened; his face radiated anger.

"I don't buy that crap. I don't buy it! If we don't help them right *here*, what's the point of our being here? How will anyone ever take us seriously?"

"But we're not set up for much!"

"We can do a heck of a lot more than just transfer! We can *do* stuff here! Guys like you give up too fast!"

I sat down wearily, shaking my head, suppressing my irritation, rubbing my eyes dazzled by the brightness of the room, and wishing over and over again I were home in bed. I did not want to get drawn into a discussion about the purpose of small country hospitals at one in the morning. I was surprised at how agitated he was, and, again, wondered what he was doing in the hospital at that hour.

"Karl, look, it's one in the morning. I'm not my best at this time. I know I'm not the ideal person to handle a really sick kid. So I plan to assess and transfer ASAP!"

Karl wagged his finger in my face, fumbling for words. Oddly, his scorn and bitterness impressed me. I wondered if I had ever been that passionate about hospitals and medicine. Karl grabbed the clipboard and waved it at me.

"Look, Einstein, I'm here already. I just happened to be here. I'll deal with this, okay? You can go home if you want."

For an instant I thought of turning around and doing just that, but my instincts stopped me. I didn't want to be upstaged. The nurses and paramedics shuffled around, in quiet and attentive pantomime, eaves-dropping and picking up every comment.

"No. I'm not going home. I'm the one on call. I don't know why you're here, but I'm glad you're here. You know more about children. You see the patient. But I'll stay and assist."

Again I wondered what he was doing in the hospital at that time in the morning. I assumed he had come to check on his patients. Karl shrugged and turned away, his voice a little softer and his body a little less stiff.

"Whatever."

"Where's the kid?" I asked. "The patient, I mean."

"I sent her for an X-ray. Five minutes."

"Five minutes, okay. Coffee?"

"Yeah."

"How do you like it?"

Karl grinned slyly.

"Just like I like my women. *Hot and black!*"

I shook my head. A couple of paramedics froze. Karl laughed. When I returned, Karl had his hands full. He was rocking a crying baby and cooing to her, making pouting faces that were grotesque and caused more wailing. The mother hovered, her eyes darting, her fingers fumbling and grasping, her grubby face contorted. She was a thin, pale woman with a smoker's face, creased and crumpled with a nervous twitch. She stood alone, unsure of herself, wearing a faded T-shirt bearing a knife and fork and the words DIXIE PIG DINER. The room reeked of urine. Karl fussed over the baby, his fingers tickling her nose and ears, his ruddy face scanning her as she twisted and screamed and searched for her mother.

"Ain't you pretty! Ain't you so *pretty!*"

Karl laid her down and reached for an infant stethoscope. Then he lifted her up again. I usually examined children that small in their mothers' arms. It was a bad sign that the baby wasn't protesting more.

"*There* now! There, there!"

I watched Karl perform his examination. He held her up to a mirror and made faces and whistled. He nodded and shook his head and eventually hummed a long crooning lullaby. The baby hesitated, then calmed down, but kept taking loud sobs and lunging for her mother. Her mother kept coming up and stroking her head, hands, and feet. Karl managed to put on the stethoscope but could not examine her. He put her down on the table and covered her with a blanket. He kept her distracted with his left hand while he tried again, this time with better luck. He listened to her heart, lungs, and abdomen. He turned her over, like a book, inspected her back, and ran his fingers down her spine, counting. He moved her head, and she gave a weak moan. He nodded and looked at me. I was impressed by Karl's diligence.

"Neck rigidity! *Definitely!*"

I repeated the exam. The girl looked weak, ill, and was experiencing neck stiffness. That raised a specter.

"So you think she's got *meningitis?*"

"Sure. Well, very likely."

Again, he examined her limbs and moved them. They hung limp and passive. She hardly moved and was rapidly becoming much quieter. He laid her down again and covered her up. As he looked at her, the baby opened her eyes and struggled to keep them open, little discs, slate gray, clouding over. She exhausted her meager resources to send one last message: looking at Karl directly she uttered a wail, like a nail scratching an empty can. Karl jumped.

"Did you hear that? *Meningitis!* She can't even cry properly! That's *bad*, real bad!"

The mother stepped forward again, shaking, and grasped Karl's forearm.

"Bin cryin all week, jes got so quiet today. I figured she was better cos she wasn't cryin', but then I sees she ain't breathin right, kind of blue lookin."

We watched the baby, her head rolling from side to side slowly, her eyes sunken and shut, her chest rising and falling erratically. Suddenly she arched herself in the bed by pushing her head and heels back in to the bed and thrusting her tiny belly upward. She held herself in a dreadful arc for a few seconds, eyes bulging, her face contorted, her upper limbs rigid with blanched fists, then abruptly went limp. Karl exploded.

"It's *got* to be meningitis!"

Her mother rushed to her and scooped her up.

"Is she real sick?"

"Yes, ma'am, she's real sick."

"How sick? Sick like she could *die?*"

"Maybe."

She gasped and clamped a hand over her mouth. She looked at me for confirmation. I nodded. Karl took the baby back, bent down, and grasped its flaccid hand, bunched it back into a fist, and patted it smartly.

"I see a vein here! Quick, get me an IV set. I'm going to start an IV here!"

The nurse, Shanna, was prepared. Shanna was large but moved with unexpected speed. Her blonde hair was pulled back tightly and stretched her round red face. She slipped on gloves and handed a pair of size nine sterile gloves to Karl. They cleaned the skin with alcohol, and Karl slid a tiny butterfly needle just below the surface. A thread of dark blood appeared in the tubing and confirmed his success.

"Dang!" Karl exclaimed.

"What's wrong, Doc?" Shanna asked.

"She didn't even flinch when I put that in!"

The mother looked at our faces in confusion, fearing the worst, scrunching up her face, leaning forward and straining to pick up any signal.

"Get me a spinal kit!"

Shanna disappeared. I pulled Karl aside and pulled him out into the corridor, not quite believing what was about to happen.

"Karl, do you think that a spinal tap is a good idea? Don't we need a CT scan first?"

"We don't have a CT scanner in this hospital, Einstein! This kid is really sick. I think she's got meningitis, and you don't need a CT scan to diagnose meningitis. You need spinal fluid, and you get that from a spinal tap. Didn't they teach you that in London?"

I ignored him, irritated by his taunts, weary and wary now that there was a concern about meningitis.

"Karl, you know that a CT is indicated to make sure there is no brain swelling before you do a spinal tap," I said. "You want to be sure there is no herniation of brain tissue when you puncture the spinal canal!"

Karl glowered, angry about the questioning.

"Look here, let me tell you something about real life medicine. *Kid's parents have no insurance.* Takes forever to get them accepted by a hospital anywhere. Maybe a teaching hospital in Dallas might take them, eventually. Maybe tomorrow or later still, okay? She's not going anywhere fast, because she's got nothing! So she needs a diagnosis right now and here and she needs a spinal tap to make the diagnosis. Are you in or are you out?"

"What if she strokes out? What if she stops breathing?" I asked, listing some of the worst-case scenarios.

"She got a snowball's chance in hell! We got to do something for her here and now! There's no time!"

"Okay, then just give her the antibiotics! Why do a spinal tap?"

"Do you not want to know what we're treating before we treat it, Einstein?"

Karl stalked back to the baby and called the mother. He washed his hands and put on sterile gloves while explaining the procedure to the mother.

"Do you understand? Your little girl may have spinal meningitis! She may have an infection of the water around the brain. We need to get your permission to do a test where we put a needle in her back and pull out a few drops of the water and check it for infection."

Her mother hesitated. She looked out the door, then closed her eyes and clasped her forehead, but said nothing. She rocked back and forth.

"She's real sick, ma'am! I told you, she could die! *Spinal meningitis!* I'm trying to help her! You want me to do this or not?"

Her mother mumbled her consent and quickly signed the forms.

Karl shot me an angry look and added, "*Read* it before you sign it, ma'am!"

She signed without reading.

Karl put on sterile gloves. Shanna peeled open the spinal tap kit and laid it out on a sterile green sheet. There was a long hollow spinal needle and an equally long thin metal rod that slid inside the needle. There was a three-way connection and a plastic tube marked out in millimeters, and a syringe, a smaller needle, and an ampoule of lidocaine. Karl turned and looked at me.

"You going to help or just sit on your ass?"

"I'll help."

"Then come here and hold the baby. I want you to curl her up real tight, put one elbow around her neck and the other around her knees. She's so small! Just curl her up real tight! I want you to make her spine bend like a high-tension bow!"

I raised the table up, pumping it with my foot, leaning forward, scooping the whimpering bundle, at first gently and then with some force, until she was tight as a balloon, the tips of her spine tenting her skin. She struggled a little in the beginning, offering enough resistance to register her unwillingness, then settled down, surrendering meekly.

Karl spun around on the stool, rapidly preparing his assault. He placed a sterile towel under her, draped green towels around her lower back, framing the lower spine. He cleaned the skin with iodine, then alcohol, then iodine again, all the time watching me, the mother and the nurse, completely in control, daring anyone to utter a word. He changed into a new pair of sterile gloves, tossing the old gloves, snatching the spinal needle, holding it up for examination, rotating it, glinting the light off its tip and finally sliding the thin metal rod into the hollow spinal needle, making it solid.

"Tighter!" Karl yelled.

I tightened further, wondering whether she could even breathe.

"You got to look for L4 and L5! You got to get into the space between L4 and L5, and I mean *exactly* into the middle of the space between L4 and L5. There's no spinal cord there, so you're safe, you're not going to hit the spinal cord."

Brakes screeched outside, and a door slammed. Moments later, a man appeared at the door. He paused, looked at Karl and then me, then the mother. He scurried to her side and tried to hold her hand. She pushed him away. The smell of alcohol became a torrent as he spoke.

"So wash the problem?"

Karl looked up. There stood before him a pale, scrawny man in jeans and a dirty vest, cigarette burns like bullet holes all over the front, glazed, gray eyes set deep in an unshaven face, staring back at him, hands now on his hips, swaying slightly.

"Wassa matta?" he asked, louder.

Karl fixed him with a look of disgust, then returned to his task. He placed two fingers of his left hand on the tips of the fourth and fifth lumbar vertebrae.

"As I was saying, you got to identify L4 and L5 and then you go *exactly* in between the two points, keeping the needle parallel to the ground."

The man glared and poked his wife.

"Wassa matta wid her?"

His wife stepped sideways. He lunged and grabbed her forearm.

"Wass the fukkin matta?"

The woman tried to peel his fingers off and looked at him with anger, starting to say something, then stopping, as if unsure whether he deserved to know. He squeezed again and she whimpered. A paramedic took a step forward. Shanna turned around and hissed.

"She's got *spinal meningitis!*"

"What?"

But Shanna had turned around. He squeezed his wife's forearm harder and she cried out. She yanked her arm out of his drunken grip and glared back at him with streaming eyes.

"She's real real sick! She got an infection in her brain, maybe! Like the nurse said! She got . . . she got . . . *smilin' mighty Jesus!*"

Karl jerked his head back and looked at her then at me with his eyes wide and mouth open in disbelief. He crossed and rolled his eyes and shook his head slowly, then returned to his task.

"Okay, nice and tight!"

I tightened. The baby whimpered. Karl selected the site, and repeated the ritual: he painted with iodine and scrubbed with alcohol. He placed his left index finger in the recess between the tips of the fourth and fifth lumbar vertebrae, then slid the index finger down to the crest of L5 and placed the middle finger on the crest of L4.

"See this tiny little space between my two fingers?" he explained to me. "You want to go exactly, and I mean *exactly*, in the middle."

He held the spinal needle, two inches long, like a thumbtack, his thumb on the base, his second and third fingers steadying the shaft. He slid it in a quarter inch, his breath held, his body tense, the fibers in his fingers sensing and relaying and analyzing the resistance. He paused briefly to exhale a little, then tensed up again and advanced the needle a fraction. The baby stiffened and yelped.

"I'm in! I'm in!"

Karl swiftly pulled the stilette, the inner metal rod, out of the needle and held a small plastic vial under the base. We waited for several seconds but no fluid emerged.

"I'm *sure* I got in! Hold on, I'm going to pull out a little!"

With exquisite care, he withdrew the needle a fraction and waited. Nothing. He mouthed *fuck* and looked up at the ceiling. He repeated the infinitesimal withdrawal and waited. He did it a fourth time. Karl looked at me with disgust and exasperation.

"Wassa matta?" asked the man, emboldened.

Nobody answered.

He took a step forward.

"Ah said, wassa matta?"

Karl pulled the needle completely out and rammed his thumb into the L4-L5 interspace. He shook his head and looked down.

"Give me another spinal needle, one size bigger. This one's a twenty-three."

"We got a twenty-one," Shanna said.

"Okay, twenty-one."

Shanna showed Karl the label and got his approval. She peeled open the package and dropped the needle onto a sterile towel. Karl snatched it up and eyed it critically, holding it up to the light, rolling it between thumb and finger, removing its stilette and sliding it back. He took a few deep breaths and swung around, his jaw clenched, his body arching, his face grim and glistening. The man stepped up to him.

"Wassa damn matta?"

The unmistakable odor of alcohol hit, a sick onion-like smell, laced with sweat and cigarette smoke. Karl looked up slowly, his hands positioned as before, his body still crouched, his voice measured.

"Who're you?" Karl asked.

"I'm the kid's dad!"

"Your kid's real sick. We got to check for a brain infection. We got to get some of the water in her spine, okay?"

"So why dint you git it already?"

"Not sure. Going to try again. Bigger needle."

The man hesitated, confused, emboldened by the recognition and wondering whether to swagger some more. He pointed a finger at Karl and opened his mouth but Karl spoke first.

"Now *shut up!*"

Karl was focused. He defined the small space again and paused, calculating, mentally mapping the depths of the ligaments between the spinous processes, and the distance between him and the spinal fluid and the best angle of entry. He licked his lips, clenched his jaw, and nodded to me. I flexed the little girl again, a rag doll, offering no resistance, folding silently in surrender. Karl held the needle parallel to the ground and slid it in, pushing on the base with tremendous calculation, moving steadily until he encountered the final resistance. Karl stopped momentarily and looked at me.

"I'm on the membrane outside the spinal canal, I'm sure of it!"

He pinched the base of the needle and left the shaft unsupported. He increased pressure on the base tangentially, recruiting muscle fibers like an orchestra raising notes. The needle quivered, then sank quickly another quarter inch. Karl exhaled and removed the stilette. We all watched and waited.

Nothing.

Karl bit his lip and pulled back a little. We watched and waited again.

Nothing.

Karl dropped his head and remained silent. I didn't know what to say. Tiredness, frustration, bewilderment, and worry sapped me, making my head heavy. My muscles quivered, and my back throbbed with pain. Sweat slipped into my eyes, stinging them, making me shake my head and try to rub them on my shoulder. An awful thought crossed my mind: What if she got worse? What if she *died?* What if she died *in my hands?*

The dad crept forward again.

"Doc!"

Karl did not look up.

"Hey, Doc!"

Karl looked up wearily.

"They's something coming out that!"

We blinked in astonishment. A drop of cloudy fluid had formed at the base of the needle and was growing before our very eyes. Before we could react, it fell on the towel and became a black spot. Karl jumped and secured the needle in position with the fingers of his left hand and held vials under the base to capture the pearly liquid. I squeezed the baby with increased vigor. Karl collected one vial, then pulled the needle back a hair. The drops came with increased frequency. The second and third vials filled up rapidly.

"We're in! *We're in!* We're in *good!*"

Karl was completely re-energized. He collected four vials of spinal fluid, then pulled the needle out with a flourish. He held the vials up to the light.

"Not a trace of blood!" he crowed.

"What do you mean?" Shanna asked.

"That means I didn't hit any blood vessels on the way in! I didn't contaminate the spinal fluid with blood!"

"Good job, Karl!" I said.

"Yeah! Thanks!"

I released my grip and straightened the baby, keeping her on her side. Karl cleaned the site again and stuck a small bandage.

"Give me some order forms! I'm going to write some admission orders! Did you see how turbid that fluid was? Meningitis!"

He stripped off his gloves and strode to the table and scribbled orders. The baby's parents looked at each other, confused but relieved. They inched forward; the mother stroked her daughter's head and the father squeezed her little fist. His eyes watered.

"Okay, Mom and Dad, she's going to be just fine," Karl explained. "I was right! She's got meningitis, but she's going to get a bunch of antibiotics and she'll be fine. Got to keep her here in the hospital."

The parents nodded wordlessly. The mother suddenly grabbed Karl's hand.

"God bless you, Doc! God *bless* you!"

Karl was flustered. He gave an awkward smile and nodded. The dad stepped forward.

"Is she really gonna to be safe here? Mebbe we best move her to Abilene."

"Look, she's going to be fine! I'm pretty sure of the diagnosis now. I think we should keep her here and start treatment. If you want to take her to Abilene, then sign her out against medical advice, and put her in your own damn car and hightail it to Abilene or wherever, it's your damn responsibility!"

The man stared at Karl suspiciously. He was debating about his answer when his wife pulled him aside and hissed in his ear. He seemed unconvinced at first but then relented, shaking his head all the while, lingering at the nurses' station, reading over again all the forms that required his signature, contesting Shanna and Karl on every clause. Karl was stern but correct, and even threw in *sir* at the end of a few explanations. Slowly, the ER cleared and I went off to wash my hands and return my coffee mug.

It was almost four a.m. when I walked to my car. The parking lot was dark, illuminated only by a distant streetlight and the ER sign. As I groped for my keys, I heard Karl cough and clear his throat. I looked back and saw him leaning against his white Chevy truck, parked opposite my Corolla. He lit a cigar and puffed.

"That took forever!"

"Yes, it did."

"Usually, my motto is, don't let your cigar burn out while you're in the ER. This time, I let it burn out. *Man*! I really think I was in the first time!"

"Maybe."

I sensed that Karl wanted to talk, so I walked over. We stood there in the dark lot, Karl drawing in deeply and exhaling luxurious clouds of blue smoke, while I slouched nearby, hands in pockets, swaying slightly from fatigue.

"Smoke bother ya?"

"No. I kinda like it."

"Want one?"

"No. Thanks."

"Whatever. More for me."

"You did a great job in there, with the spinal tap and all. I liked the way you dealt with the baby's dad."

Karl laughed.

"That idiot! Damn drunk! Bet you the reason he didn't take her to Abilene was because his liquor's here!"

"I liked the way you dealt with the mom as well."

Karl exhaled thoughtfully.

"I know something about single parents, remember? Just playing my part, y'know, the good doctor, you know. All the world's a damn stage, and the men and women merely players, right?"

I was surprised. *Shakespeare?*

"What? You think I don't know anything? Even a horse's ass like me knows some lit!"

"Didn't expect it."

"Did I ever tell you I was a semifinalist for the Rhodes scholarship?"

I was astonished.

"Don't answer. Yeah, I was the local high school hero, from a podunk little Texas town, star quarterback, good grades, rocket club, robotics, the works. Interviewed me in Dallas."

"Really! What happened?"

Karl took out his cigar and looked at me. It was his turn to look surprised.

"What do you think, Einstein? They kicked my ass out! But they were so nice to me in the interview, all polite and British and hypocritical!"

"Sorry."

"Yeah, whatever. Got to thinking about it. Even went to Oxford for a week to see what I missed. Real pretty place, pubs, parks, rivers, and all. But you know what? I figured out my philosophy of life. How to be happy."

He sucked in deeply and held it, as if imprinting his airway.

"How to be happy. The DGAS principle."

I was surrounded by a blue haze.

"What is DGAS?"

"Don't give a shit. No one really gives a shit. The scholarship people didn't give a shit. Why should I? Why should anyone? All we need is to *be happy*, who really cares about anything else? You can be happy in Hotspur; you can be happy in Oxford. Happiness is your attitude, man. So relax, don't give a shit, you don't have to impress anyone. Just gotta be happy wherever you are!"

"I like it."

"Cousin of DGAS is DGAF."

"I can figure that one out."

"Good job, Einstein! Now get you home and get some sleep!"

I jerked back, realizing where I was, peering at my watch in the dark. I mumbled a goodbye, limped to my car, and slumped. I rubbed my eyes, paused to think, found my keys, started the ignition, and inched out of the parking lot. Karl threw his lights on and honked loudly. Blinded, I slammed the brakes, and yelled. Karl bellowed.

"Seat belt and lights, Einstein! *Seat belt and lights!*"

I remained frozen. Karl honked again and again. Several households nearby woke up. I frantically strapped down my seat belt and switched the lights on. Karl finally stopped honking.

"Thus endeth the lesson! *Tiredness kills you!* Good night, Einstein!"

CHAPTER NINE

A Load on My Chest

I was startled by a scream as I walked up the ramp toward the ER. It was a clear bright morning. I had slept well the night before and felt good. I had dressed carefully and had even worn a tie. I felt I was prepared for the world. The voice rang out again, angrily.

"Get your God-damn hands off me!"

"Sparky!"

"Ferkin *useless!*"

"Sparky! Hush!"

"Get the hell outta here!"

There was a loud crash as a metal table fell to the ground and I heard glass shatter. There was an angry hubbub. I strode into the treatment room. A red-faced, middle-aged man was sitting on the edge of the gurney, an oxygen mask strapped to his face, pressing a blood-soaked piece of gauze into his left elbow. Large bandages on both hands explained his anger. He had been stuck several times, unsuccessfully, to start an intravenous line or for blood tests or both. Shanna, the nurse, recoiled in a corner, still gazing dolefully at the small dot of blood on the plastic catheter. That meant she had managed to get the tip of the needle into the vein but had not been able to advance the plastic catheter.

The man was shaking his head and glaring at Shanna. He was a short, plump man with crew-cut white hair. His denim shirt was wide open, his belly stuck out like a balloon, and a box of cigarettes peeped out of his breast pocket. He fixed a withering eye on the nurse.

"Call yourselves a firkin hospital? Can't even start a firkin IV? Hell, I should've gone to the damn vet, does a better job than you sorry bunch!"

I picked up the clipboard and read the information.

"You must be Sparky. I'm Dr. Mathur. What's the problem?"

"The problem? Can't you see? She can't start a dang IV in me!"

"Sparky, you've always been a hard stick," his wife reminded. She was a small, nervous woman with a ruddy face and black-dyed hair. Her hands trembled.

"I can see that you haven't got your IV started. But why did you come to the ER in the first place? What's the main problem? Shortness of breath?"

"Yep. Can't breathe. Been coughing and wheezing."

"You smoke too much, Sparky," hissed Shanna.

"Got nothing to do with it. *Nothing!* Don't explain why you can't start a God damn IV!"

"You really should quit!" Shanna said.

"Done it many a-time!"

He turned to me.

"Figure *you* can get it?"

"Let me try."

"You going to *try?* You any good? I've been stuck three times, I'm sick of it."

"I used to be good. When I was in London, they used to call me to start all the lines."

"I was just about to call you," Shanna explained. "Dr. Becker is on call but he won't see Sparky. He wanted me to call you."

Sparky glared at her but said nothing. He coughed up a little blood-stained sputum. His wife stepped forward.

"Let's just say him and Doc Becker got crossways with each other."

Sparky glared at her again and went into a paroxysm of coughing, ending with retching. As it ended, I approached confidently with an IV needle and a blood-pressure cuff. Sparky hacked some more and suddenly gave a huge wet cough and sprayed me with blood and phlegm. I froze in horror. Shanna suppressed a giggle. I rushed to the sink and washed my face vigorously.

"Whoa, Doc! Your white coat's a mess!"

I stripped it off.

"You got it on your shirt!"

I wiped my shirt with an alcohol swab.

"You even got it on your tie!"

I hesitated, then pulled off the tie and stared at it. It was my prized tie from the Royal College of Physicians. It was a deep blue silk tie with the Royal College emblem embossed in gold. Angry and disgusted, I threw it in the bin. I approached Sparky again with grim determination.

"Let's tie a blood-pressure cuff on his arm, and raise it above his diastolic pressure. This makes the veins really stick out."

We used his left arm. I placed the cuff over the elbow so that it would also compress the bleeding site in the elbow where he had just been stuck. I had Sparky clench and open his left hand repeatedly. I used alcohol wipes to clean an area on the forearm near the wrist. I ran the flat of my finger along the forearm and could feel the spongy linear bulge of a vein. I washed my hands and put on sterile gloves.

"This may hurt," I murmured as I cautiously advanced the tip of the needle.

There was an immediate flash of blood, and I quickly pulled out the metal stilette. Blood poured out.

"Release the cuff!"

"Are you in? Did you get it?"

"Yes."

"Ain't your first rodeo, right?"

I looked up in bewilderment. Shanna smiled.

"He means, you've done this before?"

"Yes, I have. I've used the BP cuff method before and it usually works well."

"Now what?" Sparky asked.

"Now tell me what's been happening."

"Well, Sparky's been sick for weeks," his wife explained.

"I can speak for myself, Mama."

"Well then, go right ahead, Mr. Big Shot!"

"Been sick couple three weeks. Been coughing and wheezing. This morning threw up blood."

"Did you throw it up or did you cough it up?"

"Coughed it up. Yeah, coughed it up. Anyhow, scared the shit out of me, so here I am."

"You running a fever?"

"Don't know."

"Have you coughed up blood before?"

"Yeah, a week ago."

"Sparky!" his wife said, shocked.

"How much? Would you say one or two tablespoons?"

"Yeah, about that. But main thing's the pain. Hurts real bad right here, under my tit."

"Have you been losing any weight?" I asked.

He nodded grimly and tugged at his belt buckle.

"Twenty pounds, in one month!"

I reviewed his paperwork. He was seventy, took Lisinopril for hypertension, and had no allergies.

"Have you ever had any operations? Any surgeries?"

"Appendix when I was a kid."

I wrote *appendectomy in childhood* on the form. I went over the review of systems quickly.

"Have you had any eye or sinus or skin diseases?"

"Nope."

"Any heart or lung problems?"

"He's got COPD," his wife said.

Sparky turned, but before he could say anything, he started coughing again. His face turned red and his eyes watered. Shanna handed him a paper cup of water.

"I guess I got that COPD. Been using inhalers all the time."

"Which ones? Albuterol? Steroid inhalers?"

"Yeah, both of them. Been taking steroid pills, too. *Bunch* a times."

"Any problems with severe headaches or strokes or epilepsy?"

"Nope. Man, are you going to do something or just stand there?"

"Almost done. You're not diabetic?"

"Hell no!"

He was wheezing a little with the effort of the conversation.

"Any anxiety or depression? Any anemia or low blood count problems?"

"Depressed because I live with her!"

He pointed to his wife. She smiled.

I examined him. His face and neck were flushed and swollen, with fine blood vessels visible under the pale skin of his cheeks. *Those were due to steroid therapy.* He had deep creases around his eyes and forehead, *typical of a smoker.* Hidden between those creases was an old jagged scar on the left side of his forehead. *Odd. Brain surgery?* He was sweating and his hair had started to stack. His heart sounds were obscured by his lung sounds, which were raspy and prolonged, and punctuated by showers of crackles.

"Have you had an operation on your head?"

"Oh, yeah, ah forgot. Brain tumor, been twenty years."

"Any chemo or radiation? Any recurrence?"

"Nope. On the bone, next to the brain."

Probably a meningioma, a relatively benign growth.

"Lean forward and let me check this out a little more. Take some deep breaths."

I found that the abnormal breath sounds were localized to the lower left lobe.

"Shanna, listen to the breath sounds here."

"I'm not real good with breath sounds, Doc. What should I be hearing for?"

"Normal breath sounds are a long inspiration, a pause, and then a shorter, softer exhalation. It should sound like *aaaaaaah-huuh*. But he has bronchial breathing over the left lower lobe. The exhalation is much longer, almost as long as the inhalation, and quite loud, sounds like *aaah-aaaaah*. It means there could be an infection in that area. Listen!"

She listened, but wasn't impressed.

"Let's get an X-ray."

Sparky peeled off his shirt. He had a barrel-shaped chest, large breasts and a protuberant belly. *Large breasts in a male? That's unusual. It could be benign, but it could be due to something sinister, like alcoholic liver disease or lung cancer.* He lifted up his right breast.

"You got to see this thing!"

There was a hard lump under the skin, about the size of a walnut, lifting up his right nipple. The skin slid over it but the lump did not move from side to side and was firmly attached to the underlying rib.

"I don't like that," I said slowly straightening up.

"Why not?"

"Bothers me. I'll tell you later, but I think we should biopsy it."

The rest of the examination was unremarkable. Sparky started coughing again. Prolonged wheezing followed this fit.

"Okay, let's get him some breathing treatments. Half a cc of albuterol in two cc of normal saline, repeat in a couple of hours. And give him Solumedrol sixty mg IV now. Is he on antibiotics?"

"No, Doctor," Shanna responded.

"Let's see the X-ray before we decide anything else."

I turned to Sparky.

"Sparky, you're too weak to go home. You need to be admitted. I can make arrangements to send you to Abilene, or if you prefer, we could keep you here. Whatever you want, but you can't go home."

"Doc, what do you recommend?" Sparky's wife asked.

"Transfer to Abilene."

"Hell, no! I ain't going nowhere! Give me a shot and let me go!"

"Sparky, *listen* to the man! He's saying you got to go into the hospital."

"I can call the specialists at Abilene Regional Hospital. That's the closest big hospital."

"Hell, no! That's where Travis died! I ain't going there."

"You can't go home like this! Would you like me to go ahead and admit you here? Or call another hospital?"

Sparky looked helplessly at his wife, who nodded encouragingly. He looked at the floor, then burst into another paroxysm of coughing. This one ended with him collecting sputum in his mouth. He spat it out on paper tissue and held it up for me to see. It was streaked with bright red blood.

"Okay," he croaked. "Okay. I'll stay here. But I got a condition."

"What's that?"

"You've got to let me *have my cigarettes*. You'll let me have my cigarettes?"

I didn't know what to say. I looked away and busied myself in paperwork.

"Doc, I need an answer! Will you let me have my cigarettes?"

I looked back at him. He looked defiant, even though he was struggling to breathe and was muzzled with an oxygen mask. I was irritated by his attitude, I was irritated by his refusal to be transferred, and I was irritated about losing my tie. I glanced at the bin. *Retrieve the tie?*

"Will you let me have my cigarettes?"

Maybe I could fish it out when nobody's looking.

"Doc, *will you let me have my cigarettes*?"

"All right!"

I ignored Shanna's shocked expression. The laboratory technician, Joe, walked in and wordlessly jammed a wet X-ray film on the viewing box. He turned it on and appraised the film.

"Don't look good t'me. What d'you think, Doc?" Joe asked.

I examined it carefully. *I better not miss anything.*

119

"There's a lot of information here. Look at the lung shadows. They're supposed to be two big black cylinders on both sides of the heart."

"Doesn't look black to me," Sparky said.

"You're right. They're mottled white and they are actually too big. That's called hyperinflation, and it happens because air gets trapped in his lungs. He can suck air in but he can't push it out. So he has mottled, hyperinflated lungs and that tells us he has COPD, chronic obstructive pulmonary disease."

"I coulda tole you that," croaked Sparky, unimpressed.

"But here's the problem. See this white area in the bottom of the left lung? This is due to consolidation or thickening and is probably due to pneumonia."

"So you were right," Shanna said. "He does have pneumonia."

There were other features that I did not discuss. The main airway is the trachea and it was pulled *toward* the pneumonia. Normally, pneumonia causes the tissues to bulge and pushes the trachea *away* or leaves it midline. So if the trachea was being pulled toward the pneumonia, then there was probably something causing that tissue to shrink and pull the trachea *toward* it. That *thing* could well be a cancer, especially in a smoker.

And there was that area on the right eighth rib, that lump that was attached to the rib but not to the skin. Half an inch of the upper-rib margin was eroded, wiped away as if with an eraser. This was bad news. These were the features of a cancer, probably metastatic, and the primary was probably in the left lower lobe, causing collapse and pneumonia. The X-ray could mean advanced lung cancer.

"I'm writing his admission orders, Shanna. Sparky, I need to talk to you and your wife later today, once you feel better. Right now, we need to get your breathing sorted out. Go ahead and take him to the floor, I'll bring you the orders."

Later, once I was alone, I fished out my tie. I folded it and slipped it inside a red, plastic biohazard bag and thought, *Do I need to tell the dry cleaner?*

I wrote the admission orders and left them at the nurses' station. I went into Sparky's room and explained the plans to him and his wife and went upstairs to the clinic.

There was no one for me to see that morning, so I retired to the break room and took out my *Complete Guide to the Internal Medicine Board Examination*, and selected the section on lung diseases. Before long, I came across a passage.

You have a sixty-year-old bricklayer, a two-pack-a-day smoker. He presents with a month's history of coughing and wheezing. The exam shows crackles in the right base and the X-ray is shown below. After initial care, what is the next best step?

The X-ray showed the right-sided consolidation and the trachea pulled to that side. I looked at the choices. The right answer was *Bronchoscopy*. Bronchoscopy is a procedure in which a very thin flexible fiber-optic tube is passed into the trachea. The inner lining of the trachea and its branches, the right and left bronchi, can be seen on a TV screen. A channel in the tube allows the passage of a long, slender biopsy forceps, which can obtain tiny pieces of suspicious tissue. Sparky would *have* to go to Abilene and see a specialist. I decided to see him after lunch and insist on it.

Sparky looked a lot better that afternoon. He was sitting up in bed, taking a breathing treatment when I walked in. His wife was standing beside him, mopping his face. He coughed a greeting and pushed her aside.

"Feelin much better, Doc!"

"You look better."

"Can ah go home?"

"I don't think so. You're still pretty weak."

I sat down on the side of the bed and looked at him.

"Sparky, I'm worried about you. I know you have pneumonia, and you have COPD, and we're treating you for it. But I'm worried that there may be something else."

"Like what? Cancer?"

I was taken aback. I mumbled.

"Well, yes, that's possible. The best way to find out is to send you to Abilene and have them do a test called bronchoscopy."

"Hell, no. Already tol' ya, Doc. Ain't happenin."

"Sparky, we have to find out what's going on in your chest!"

"Ain't happening. Ain't goin."

I looked at his wife, pleading.

"No sense talking t'me. He don't lissen a word what I say."

"You don't have to make a decision right away. Think about it."

"Ain't changing nuthin. Ain't goin, period."

I stood up, defeated.

"There is one other option. I can take a biopsy of the lump on your chest."

Sparky and his wife looked at each other. Sparky nodded.

"You kin do it here? Ah'm game fir thet."

I had Shanna come and assist me. It was a simple procedure. With Sparky lying down, I quickly cleaned the area around his right breast with iodine and alcohol. It dried rapidly. I slipped on sterile gloves and injected two percent lidocaine into the skin immediately above, below, to the right and to the left of the lump, creating small blisters. I injected slowly to reduce the pain of injection. A few minutes later, the lump was numb.

I grasped a scalpel and made a small X-shaped incision at the vertex and mopped the bead of blood that immediately welled up. After a few seconds of pressure, I lifted the gauze. Granular yellow tissue bulged.

"Looks like grits," Shanna declared.

"Cancer?" asked Sparky.

"Oh, we can't tell just by looking. I'm going to take a tiny piece and I'll send it to the lab. Does it hurt?"

"Nah, don hurt."

I used the tip of the scalpel to cut out three small blocks of tissue and put them in a sterile container containing formalin, a preservative. I wrote Sparky's full name and date of birth and the date of the collection and turned it over to Shanna.

"Will that cost extra, Doc?" his wife asked.

"I don't know. We need some answers here. I tried to get Sparky to go to Abilene but he refused, so we're doing the next best thing."

"Sparky, you should listen to the doctor!" his wife said.

Sparky shook his head and didn't answer. I busied myself, putting a bandage on the biopsy site. It looked clean.

"I wan mah ciggrets now. I've done the boppsy."

Sparky staggered to his feet, half-helped, half-hindered by his wife. He was trying to get to the box of cigarettes on the table by the door.

"Sit down, Sparky!" I said.

"Hell, no. Ah wan mah ciggrets!"

He lunged forward and the IV pole came crashing down. Sparky fell back on the bed. The clamor drew in another nurse, and she stepped forward to restrain him. He swung at her and missed.

"Ferkin sheyt!"

"Call security!" I ordered, trying to sound calm and firm.

"We don't have security. Get Joe from the lab!" the nurse called out. Sparky drew himself up on his IV pole and pointed at me wrathfully. "You promised me! You promised ah could have mah ciggrets!" I was speechless. "You *firkin* promised!"

He was racked by coughing and doubled over. He reached out for tissue and held it to his mouth and rapidly soaked it with thick green sputum streaked with blood. This lasted minutes. Eventually, he straightened himself and glared, still gasping for breath. He seemed to be summoning the strength to repeat everything. Instead of sitting down, he lunged for his cigarettes and fell short. I swung back angrily to the table and snatched the pack. I thrust them onto his chest. He grabbed them in astonishment and sat down.

"Here! You can *have* them!"

He looked up at me victoriously.

"You can *have* them, I *promised* you that. But you can't *smoke* them!"

An incredulous look made its way across his face. His mouth opened. He looked at his wife and back at me. He shook his head slowly.

"Ah kin *have* 'em but ah can't *smoke* 'em! Ah got a firkin *wiseguy* ez mah doctor!"

He sat down. He started laughing, and the staff joined in. I turned and walked out. As I left, I heard him say, "You a firkin *wiseguy*, thas what! Firkin *wiseguy!*"

He laughed again and resumed coughing.

CHAPTER TEN

Friday Football:
The Hail Mary Pass

As Karl said, football is the state religion of Texas. National, college, and high school football is attended, debated, celebrated, and venerated like no other sport. In small towns, the high school football coach is often more important than the mayor. High school football matches are played Friday nights during fall and winter. Hotspur High School had the Spur Cats, and their blue-and-white logo adorned every business on Commercial Avenue and almost every car and truck in town. On Fridays, the cougar's head emblem would pop up on faces, foreheads, and wrists, and in tempera on cheeks and deltoids. Everyone wore jeans and blue-and-white-striped shirts and headbands. Folks huddled on the streets and in the drugstores and in the post office, discussing the players and the tactics and the odds.

At nine in the morning, everyone went to the high school gym for the pep rally, a boisterous gathering of all the high school students and the able-bodied citizenry, marshaled by the teachers and whipped up into a frenzy by the school band. I had no idea about this ritual when I first joined, so I found myself in a deserted clinic on a Friday morning in November, around ten o'clock, along with two sullen members of the office staff. Dr. Becker was the football team doctor and left early for the rallies. Two of his sons were on the team; his older, a junior, was being groomed for quarterback. I sat and drained my second cup of coffee, glanced over the pages of Karl's *Guns and Ammo*, and scanned the empty waiting room. I feigned interest in the magazine, trying to ignore the fact that I was such an outsider. The phones rang but the staff ignored them, gazing into the distance, not even bothering to look up or at each other. Their dogged petulance amused and irritated me. I flung down my magazine and reached for the phone.

Before I could pick it up, the door of the waiting room burst open and Gideon Gerhart, an ER nurse, burst in, his face flushed with excitement. He hurtled to the check-in window and pounded the counter.

"What in *hell's name* is wrong with y'all?" he demanded. "Why ain't y'all answering the *damn phone?* Where's the doctor?"

I rose to my feet.

"Doc, we *need* you downstairs in the ER right now and I mean, *right now!* We got a real sick patient and he's fixin' to *explode!*"

We raced out. I felt a surge of guilt: I had allowed the staff to slack off. We flew down the stairs, two steps at a time, past the astonished pink ladies and the lab phlebotomists. The word *explode* stuck in my mind, and I racked my mind to short-list medical conditions that could possibly present that way.

There were several people outside the ER and we blazed past them. In the ER an enormous man with a mop of sopping wet blond hair sat straddling the examination table as if it were a horse, his head turned sharply to his left side. The right side of his neck was swollen to twice the normal size and was the reason his head was pushed over so force-fully. His face was turning blue, bathed in sweat; his eyes bulged and his mouth gasped and gulped. His shirt was ripped open and his chest heaved. He leaned forward, arms straight and hands clamped on his knees, and rocked unsteadily. The heart leads, loosened by sweat, were on the verge of falling off. Gideon pushed them back on and turned to me. He was a small, thin, nervous man, bald, with round glasses. He looked like a white Gandhi.

"What in *Sam Hill* are we gonna do, Doc? What are we *gonna do?*"

I stood, astonished.

"Who is this?" I asked.

A petite lady offered her hand.

"Sir, this is my husband, Cactus Leftwich. He's a rancher. He can't talk right now, sir."

Cactus tried to say something and collapsed in a spasm. He clutched at his throat. The oxygen tubing snapped off and fell to the ground; he lunged for it and almost fell. I jumped to his side.

"Quick, get him oxygen by face mask! Now! Turn it up to fifty percent and put on the pulse ox and get the EKG leads on him! Get the X-ray tech in here now and get me a stat chest film, and get me a blood gas!"

"Resp'tory tech's a gone right now, Doc!" Gideon said.

"What?"

"School. Pep rally."

"Give me the syringe, I'll draw it myself!"

"I don't know where he left the blood gas syringes, Doc! I'm sorry!"

"Just give me a five cc syringe with half a cc of heparin, that'll do."

I listened to his chest carefully. There were good breath sounds on the left and rapid heart sounds, but nothing on the right. I listened again, closely, holding my breath. Nothing. I heard no breath sounds at all. I listened carefully to the back of his chest as well. No breath sounds on the right side. It seemed that air was trapped in his right lung. I laid the fingers of my left hand flat against the chest wall, in the spaces between his ribs, and tapped on them with my right middle finger, a technique called percussion. The chest cavity resounded like a drum on the right side. I checked the left side for comparison. Normal.

I palpated the trachea, the windpipe with Adam's apple sticking out in front. The trachea is always in the midline, but, in his case, it was pushed over to the left side. Cactus was tiring and sagged. Gideon helped me.

"You checking his trachea?"

"Yes."

"Deviated to the left?"

"Yes."

"So what does that mean?"

"That means that something on the right side is pushing it over to the left."

"I've seen it before with a pneumo!"

"Yes, it could be a right-sided pneumothorax."

I palpated the chest wall and felt crackling. I could feel small bubbles of air underneath the skin, and they shifted and popped under the weight of my palm like bubble wrap. The right side of the neck had the same sickening feel. I recoiled in shock.

"He's got crepitus!"

"What's that?" Gideon asked.

"He's got air creeping in under his skin! It *must* be a pneumothorax!"

"A what?"

"A pneumothorax! The right lung has probably collapsed and is leaking air into his right chest and from there to his neck. We need that X-ray now!"

His wife inserted herself in front of me.

"You know, he had that, once before. About ten years ago. Even had it once when he was in high school, playing football."

"Running back," Cactus whispered. "I was running back."

"He's a football legend, Doc! He played for Texas and for the Cowboys!"

I didn't realize how important that was.

"We need an X-ray, stat!"

"I don't know if he's here, Doc!'

I stared in bewilderment. Gideon shrugged.

"I'll get him here pronto, Doc! Here's your blood gas syringe, I put the heparin in it."

He shot out to find the X-ray technician. *The pep rally? I really needed the X-ray to make the diagnosis!*

I started Cactus on oxygen by facemask and he settled down a little. It gave me seconds to think. *Am I right? Is this really crepitus?* I reflected on the time I had felt crepitus before, in London, when I was in training. A young woman had been in a car wreck and the side of her neck had felt like bubble wrap. It had felt crackly, like this. *But is it really crepitus? It has to be! It made sense, and was compatible with the other findings. Could he have done something to collapse his lung on the right side and that had allowed air to track into his neck?* I looked at Cactus's neck again. To my horror, it had swollen up even more. The air was accumulating ever more rapidly, and, with every breath, he was trapping more air in his right lung and compressing his trachea and his left lung.

I thought of intubating Cactus, putting a plastic tube into his airway to move air in and out more efficiently. However, that would run the risk of pushing even more air into his right lung and into his neck, and make him worse. He was deteriorating, and could collapse and die in minutes! I looked at him, my heart pounding. His slate eyes stared back, scared, but steady. I looked down, hiding my panic. I thought of London and Houston, and how I had dealt with sick patients before. But I was alone here, again. Where was the rest of the team? Where was the X-ray? He could die! I desperately needed the X-ray.

Calm down, I told myself. *Calm down. Breathe.*

Okay, in London, as team leader, I would order a stat chest X-ray and get an arterial blood gas. The X-ray tech is coming. But I need to get the arterial blood sample myself.

I squatted down on a stool and pulled up a surgical tray. I opened a pack of iodine swabs and slipped on surgical gloves. His wristwatch was on his left wrist, which meant he probably was right-handed. Normally, I would have tried the left wrist so as to spare the dominant side, but there was no time and the right side was going to be easier for me anyhow. I could not risk missing the artery. I grasped his right wrist and painted it quickly with two layers of iodine and blew on it gently to dry it up. I knocked the cap off the needle and held the heparinized syringe like a pen in my right hand. I quickly isolated the radial artery between the tips of two left fingers and separated the tips a fraction, stretching the skin. Holding the syringe at an angle, I slid it down in that space, advancing very cautiously, just a few millimeters, and not daring to breathe.

"Big stick now!" I yelled out, after the event.

But Cactus did not notice. Abruptly, the syringe jerked to life and crimson burst into the syringe, lifting the plunger with its pressure. The whole syringe jerked synchronously with his heartbeat. This was definitely an arterial stick. I let three milliliters in and then pulled out the syringe, pressing down on the site with great force. I rolled the syringe on my thigh to mix it with the heparin to prevent it from clotting, then held it up and cried out.

"*Hey!* This is the sample for the blood gas! Get this to the lab now! *Right now!*"

"Okay, Doc!" Gideon responded.

"And get me some cotton swabs and a pressure dressing for the radial artery! We need pressure on this site. Where's the tech?"

Gideon's face gave me the answer.

"I called him in, Doc. He's coming in fast as he can!"

I stood up and looked at Cactus. Yes, the neck was getting bigger. He was still struggling, but his heaving was less forceful. *Less forceful. That's a bad sign! He's getting tired, and that means he may stop breathing!* I glanced again at the monitor. Oxygen saturation ninety percent, occasionally dropping to eighty-eight percent, heart rate one hundred and fifty-five to one hundred and sixty, blood pressure ninety by sixty, and dropping.

He's not going to make it, I thought. *What could I do? He's going to die, right here, right now!*

Gideon handed me the blood gas report. His oxygen and carbon dioxide levels were low, as I expected, but I was alarmed to find that his pH was normal.

"I thought you would be happy that at least his pH was normal," Gideon murmured. Cactus's wife moved closer, unable to sit still, kneading her husband's hat.

"He's breathing so fast, he should be blowing off his CO_2 and his pH should be high rather than normal or low. The fact that the pH is normal means he's *not* keeping up. He's getting exhausted and isn't compensating," I whispered back.

Cactus was listing badly. His chest rose and fell mightily, but the cadence was slowing and the breathing was becoming shallow. He looked like a rider about to fall off his horse. I couldn't wait any longer.

"Get me a hundred cc syringe with an eighteen-gauge needle!"

"With what in it?"

"Nothing. Nothing. Empty!"

"Nothing? Nothing at all?"

"Just get it, okay?"

If there was air trapped in the right chest cavity, I had to let it out. I decided to use the syringe to find out if there was air in the chest by trying to suck some out. If there were air under pressure, then the syringe would fill up rapidly. If I was wrong, then there would be no air, or, worse, *I would puncture the lung and possibly push him over the edge myself.* He was getting quieter and his blood gas report confirmed that he was getting tired. He could collapse and go into cardiac arrest if I waited. *But there was still no chest X-ray.* And there was no time.

"Get his wife to sign a consent for a chest tube! I'll explain it to her! Get her to the door!"

I pulled over the tray again and positioned it closer to his chest. I sat down and pulled on fresh gloves.

"Give me some lidocaine and a ten cc syringe!"

Gideon placed a fresh green surgical towel on the tray and peeled open a syringe and needle and dropped them on the tray, taking care to avoid touching the tray, maintaining sterility. He cracked open an ampoule of lidocaine and held it open. I tried to get closer on the stool and bumped into the tray, knocking down the syringe and needle.

"Damn it! *Damn it!*" I cried out, before I could contain myself.

I looked up and saw his wife standing there, scared and silent. I realized, for the first time, that she was a beautiful woman, careful hair, clean features, filmy eyes, and soft wrinkles, clad in jeans and a bright blue-and-white-striped shirt and a headband that said *Go Spur Cats*. She had one hand over her mouth and the other on the table for support. She trembled, then steadied herself and spoke.

"Doctor, I don't think I introduced myself properly. I'm his wife, Geneva. What do I need to sign? What's this for?"

"Ma'am, I think Cactus has got a lot of air trapped in his chest, and it's pressing on his lungs, so he can't breathe. I want to check so I want to put in a needle and drain the air out of him—I mean, out of his chest."

She grasped my elbow.

"You do what you got to do, Doc. You have my permission. God bless you!"

"Thanks," I mumbled, still embarrassed.

I looked at the chest wall and selected a site. *Not too low now, or I'll puncture the liver. Somewhere here, in between the eighth and tenth ribs, that should do it.* I nervously counted down the ribs and selected a spot on the side, below the armpit, in between the eighth and ninth ribs. I cleaned it rapidly with iodine and loaded up a fresh syringe with lidocaine.

"I'm just numbing it up now," I explained to Cactus, slowly injecting the lidocaine under the skin and raising a blister. I then injected at a deeper level and then deeper still. Cactus didn't wince. I discarded the small syringe and picked up the large one hundred cc syringe. I held my breath for a second, and thought again. *What if I puncture his lung?*

"*Trust* you, Doc!" Cactus gasped.

"Cactus, I'm going to try to get the air out of your chest. You may feel some pain as I go in, okay?"

Cactus grunted, barely. I emptied the syringe by pushing the plunger all the way down. I gritted my teeth and guided the tip of the needle into the chest cavity. I hoped that the pressure of the trapped air would push up the plunger immediately, proving that there was compressed air. But nothing happened. I moved the whole assembly forward and backward a little. Nothing. I pulled the whole needle out and slid it in again, at a different angle. Again, nothing. I could tell by the lack of resistance that I was in the chest cavity, but nothing was happening to the plunger in the syringe. Was I wrong? Was he suffering from something else? Had I *punctured his lung?* My mouth dried up and my tongue turned numb, signs I always experience on the cusp of some awful realization.

Maybe I missed the diagnosis! What if I just made him worse?

I had nothing to lose. I was already in too deep, literally. I gently pulled on the plunger. It came back remarkably smoothly. I pulled a little more. It obliged again. I was suddenly hopeful.

"You feel anything? Any better?"

I looked up hopefully. Cactus looked down, still sweating, head still turned to the left, and shook his head. His wife began to sniff. Gideon moved to comfort her. I steeled myself and pulled the plunger back completely, pulling out a hundred cc of air and then pulled the syringe completely out. I pushed out the air, and with an air of defiance, plunged the needle in again in the same place and pulled out another syringeful of air. Again, it came out easily. Again, Cactus felt no better. I did it a third time.

"Any better?"

This time, he hesitated. I looked at the monitor. As I watched, his heart rate decreased, from one hundred and sixty per minute to one hundred and forty-five per minute. His oxygen saturation picked up a little to ninety-two percent.

Cactus managed a weak grin and winked.

I pulled out a total of nine hundred cc before Joe, the X-ray technician, came bursting in, and we all stood aside for the X-ray. He was wearing jeans and a striped shirt emblazoned with a lightning bolt and GO SPUR CATS! I noted with satisfaction that Cactus was able to co-operate by leaning backward as the X-ray film was placed behind his chest and the beam was aligned. Joe scooped up the film cassette and left the X-ray machine in the room in case another exposure was needed. Cactus smiled at us, but seemed exhausted by the effort. His wife wiped his wet forehead and kissed it, murmuring and reassuring.

Joe came back, breathless.

"Here it is, Doc!"

He thrust the wet film onto the view box. There was no mistaking it, a huge pneumothorax on the right side with air tracking up under the skin of the neck on the right side. I was so relieved I could have cried. I said nothing, and, with effort, remained calm.

"*Son of a gun!*" Gideon whooped. "Pneumothorax! Pneumothorax! *Goddamn* pneumothorax!"

I ordered a chest drain and put on a gown and fresh gloves. I numbed up the skin again and placed a larger needle in the chest cavity, and then exchanged it for a soft plastic tube that snaked into the chest cavity but hung down limply inside close to the wall and would not scratch the lung as it reinflated. I stitched it into place and connected it to a collecting apparatus, which contained a water seal to prevent air from flowing the wrong way. I noted with satisfaction the air collecting there, bubbling through the water. I looked up again, into Cactus's face and saw that he was swallowing hard and repeatedly.

"Mouth's real dry, Doc," he croaked. "Water?"

"Yes, yes, of course."

Gideon handed him a cup of tap water, and he gulped it down and handed it back for more. Gideon gave him two more refills. Cactus winked at me again and smiled. He nodded to indicate *I'm better*, but saved his energy for breathing. His wife wiped his face and his arms, and he changed positions, finally settling down hunched over the end of the gurney, sucking deep draughts from the oxygen mask. His wife gave me a thumbs-up.

Gideon wheeled around.

"Doc, I forgot. Your wife's been trying to reach you. You need to call her."

Cactus looked better. I didn't want to tie up the phone in the room so I stepped into the anteroom. I could look out through the door and keep an eye on Cactus.

"Hi, Maya! Sorry, I was tied up!"

"No problem. I just wanted to tell you something," she hesitated and went on. "You know, I was at the grocery store, getting the food for the dinner tonight. You remember, I had invited the Coopers for dinner?"

"Oh, now I remember. I had forgotten."

"They hadn't answered. I went to the grocery store and there was a problem with the credit card. It wouldn't go through. But the manager said he knew you and made some calls, it got sorted out, and I went home."

"Maybe we didn't pay in time?"

"Well, I got home and Mr. Cooper called me. He's the bank manager, I didn't know that, but anyway, he called me and was very polite and asked that you call him."

"Why?"

"I don't know. Something to do with our account or maybe the credit card. And when I said, 'Well, we'll see you tonight,' he was really strange and didn't seem to acknowledge that he was coming."

"I'll call him."

"And then call me back and tell me what's going on."

"Of course."

While talking to Maya, I saw Karl burst into the room. He, too, was wearing blue jeans and a striped Spur Cats shirt. He stood still for a moment and took it all in. Then he plunged forward, hugged the wife, slapped Cactus on his good shoulder and greeted him warmly, back-kicked a stool, sat on it, and started examining the chest tube minutely. I signed off and rushed back, both grateful and resentful to see Karl.

"*Whoa!* You put in a *chest tube!*"

"Yeah. He had a tension pneumothorax," I said, trying to sound nonchalant.

"Tension pneumo! *Sweet Jesus!*"

"But he's stable now. His O-two sats are close to a hundred percent."

Karl swarmed all over Cactus. He asked questions, examined the chest, tugged on the chest tube, and reviewed the labs.

"Man! You put in a *chest tube!*"

"Pneumos often recur."

"Yeah. Still, pretty risky. You pulled air out his lung without an X-ray? Good call, though. You know what we call that in Texas?"

"No."

"We call that a Hail Mary pass. You do some big play like throw the football all the way to the end zone and you say a prayer that one of your guys grabs it!"

"You mean, taking a big chance."

"Yep."

He turned.

"How you feeling, Cactus?"

Cactus nodded and gave him a thumbs-up.

"Yeah, he looks ready for transfer. You called anyone?"

"No, I haven't had the time. You know someone I should call?"

"Don't worry about it. I'll take care of it. I'll call David Stryker in Abilene. We went to med school together. He's my buddy. I'll ship him. I'll take it from here."

I stood there, unsure of what to do next. I felt that my glory was being stolen. *Karl wants to be Citizen of the Year, that's why.* I was about to protest when Karl continued.

"Hey, you better go to Admin. They got a phone call for you from your bank."

I was astonished. All concerns about fame and glory vanished, and I remembered what Maya had just said. *Bank troubles? Had we overdrawn? Are we low on cash? Why is the bank calling me in the hospital?* I stammered my goodbyes to Cactus and his wife and rushed off. I found Francisca conducting a tranquil conversation on the phone. She waved me to the sofa and indicated *one minute.* I could not sit down and paced in front of her desk. She covered the mouthpiece and whispered *It's for you!* and went back to the conversation. Finally she nodded vigorously and chuckled and said goodbye. She thrust the phone toward me and said brightly, "It's for you, Dr. Mathur!"

"Hey, Doc! How are you? This is Buddy Cooper at the bank! You got a minute?"

"Sure."

I looked at Francisca and wished she wasn't there. She smiled back and looked at me blankly. She listened happily to every word.

"Doc, I wanted to tell you that my wife, Allison Sue, saw your wife, Maya, in the grocery store. She told me your wife had a problem with her credit card. Then Les Greenway, the store manager, called me."

I flushed.

"Well, maybe I didn't pay the bill in time."

"Yeah, you didn't. Anyhow, I got to looking at your balance and you sure are running low!"

I didn't know what to say.

"So I thought I might tell you that you should be getting almost a thousand dollars from the hospital for every weekend you covered the ER."

"*Really?*"

"Now that they're finally getting paid by Medicare!"

Francisca was nodding and rummaging in her desk.

"You covered six weekends so they owe you about six thousand, Doc! Come on by and deposit it and you'll be just fine!"

I struggled.

"How did you know all this?"

"I was at the pep rally and Allison Sue met Betty Becker, and they were just talking and I remembered that the hospital hadn't paid you your salary, but it had paid the other docs for the weekends, so I figured they had enough to pay you as well! So I checked with Francisca who was right there in the school parking lot and sure enough! You got a few checks sitting there!"

A wave of relief came over me.

"That's great!"

"So pick them up and hurry on over! Remember, we close early today! It's Friday!"

"Will do."

"One more thing. Thank you for looking after Cactus. He's kin to me, distant, but kin nevertheless, and what's more, he's a good man and he goes to my church."

"How did you know about Cactus?"

"Lab tech Joe Fastow was there at the pep rally and he got called back to do the X-ray. He told us Cactus was in the ER. Then I just kind of called around. I got to thinking about you and talking to folks about you! Remembered what Allison Sue had just said about your wife's credit card getting rejected. All worked out for you!"

"Thanks!"

"You know Cactus played for Texas and for the *Dallas Cowboys*? Practically *royalty* round here."

"I just found out."

"We'll see you at the game tonight?"

"You're not coming for dinner?"

"Dinner? On a *Friday* night? Doc, that's impossible! I figured you were joking or something!"

"Maybe some other time."

"Sure, we can have dinner any day but Friday. Friday's football! Hey, good job, Doc! See you!"

I hung up. Francisca smiled and handed me an envelope.

"Cactus just took over from Coach Johnson as hospital board president. In fact, he's on every board in town! Everyone loves him."

As I left she added a postscript.

"It's a really good thing he didn't die here! *Hospital Board President Dies in His Own ER* is what the Dallas paper would have said!"

The ER was full of people wearing jeans and striped shirts. They talked with Cactus and patted him on the shoulder and shook his hand. They smiled and waved to me. Cactus was strapped into a gurney and the paramedics swarmed all over him. Karl ordered them about. I watched from the door, then left.

———————

Cactus's wife called later that night.

"He's still in surgery. Dr. Stryker is doing the surgery. Dr. Karl arranged it all. The surgeon was waiting for us when we got here and they got him straight in."

"That's great! I hope he does well."

"Doc, I just wanted to say thank you."

"You're welcome."

"I have to go now, but thank you. You pulled him through, Doc. I told all my family, he wouldn't be here if it weren't for you."

"I'm glad I could help."

"God bless."

Later, as I was trying to fall asleep, I turned the day's events over in my head.

He wouldn't be here if it weren't for you.

I replayed it over and over. It felt wonderful.

It's the best part of medicine.

I thought of medical school, of residency, of fellowship, of research, of the convoluted path my life had taken. India, Bahrain, London, Houston, Hotspur. I had seen so much life and death in training, in big city hospitals, rising up the ranks, slowly improving my art. I remembered my mentors, my failures and successes, and how so many years had condensed into the ultimate measure: *experience*.

I had completed my training, passed my exams, but always had a nagging concern. *Am I ready? Am I really capable?* In a dusty corner of Texas, in a small ER, without a safety net, I finally convinced myself: *I was as ready as I would ever be.*

CHAPTER ELEVEN

Impaled

We were getting ready for breakfast. I had *Sesame Street* on again, milk and cereal out, and waffles in the toaster. OJ Simpson had just been acquitted, and the sensational news had overwhelmed the airwaves. The nation was in an uproar, and the world was following along, but here, in our home, Big Bird was the biggest character around, and the only debate at that moment was whether to switch to *Barney the Friendly Dinosaur* or stay with the rerun.

I looked out the kitchen window at the brush beyond the fence. The sun had risen, and the mesquite trees, the stubby bushes, and the thorny mesquites behind our house were starting to gleam. Blue jays sailed around the dry birdbath. I watched them glumly.

"Still not enough patients in the clinic?" Maya asked, collecting the waffles.

"No."

"Maybe some will show up later."

"Maybe."

"Got to have a positive attitude, right?"

I was silent.

"Positive attitude, right?"

"Yeah, positive attitude. Right."

I turned away. I thought about what the cable guy had said. *I don't know if you can make it here, Doc.*

"Priya! Anjali! Breakfast!" I yelled.

"If you go to work with that kind of attitude, no one will *want* to see you!"

I thought about that.

"I guess so. I'll feel better later."

After breakfast, I drove off in my old red Corolla. I drove past the neat new houses on the hill, with their manicured yards, down the hill, past the older residences with red brick and thick white mortar and wide swaths of St. Augustine grass, and finally on Nueces past crumbling two- and three-room buildings with peeling paint, broken windows, and cars on blocks in front. I drove past a cross on the side of the road, festooned with blue and white bunting and school badges. I coasted into the hospital and parked near the Emergency Room. Dr. Becker's big white Chevy truck was already there, parked near the clinic. *He's already seeing patients,* I thought enviously. I went to chat with the ER staff before starting my vigil in the clinic. I had begun to know the staff well and felt at home. Gideon Gerhart greeted me warmly.

"Cactus was on the news last night. No new taxes!"

"Great!"

"Hear about OJ?"

"Yes, of course. But what's happening here?"

"Nothing yet, but there was something on the police scanner," Gideon said, wiping his round glasses. "Some deal at Lancaster Manufacturing."

"What kind of problem?" I asked.

"Don't know. I'll call you," Gideon promised.

"How's your wife?"

"Good, good. Thanks for asking. Get you some coffee, Doc?"

"Thanks, I'll get it upstairs."

I walked past the administration counter and waved at Francisca, who blew me a kiss. I chatted with the pink ladies setting up shop under the stairs, and even wished Joe in the lab a good morning.

Better attitude, that's the key. Laugh, and the world laughs with you.

I ambled up the two flights of stairs to the clinic upstairs. I entered through the side door and was greeted by a gale of general chaos and hilarity. Everyone was talking excitedly except Heather, the office manager, who sat stiffly at her desk, looking resolutely at her screen. She was a pleasant forty-year-old brunette with a soft nose and keen black eyes. Heather wore her glasses low on her nose and had her hair in a tight bun. She spoke without looking up, her lips pursed in disapproval.

"Watch out, Dr. Mathur," Heather warned me. "It's Dr. Becker. He's got a new *toy*."

"What kind of toy?"

"Oh, you'll find out soon enough."

I poured myself some coffee and looked around. Karl was nowhere. I presumed he was with a patient. There were a few patients in the waiting room. I sidled over to Amber, the reception and appointment clerk. She was a slender blonde, with long silky hair that dropped in pretty bangs and curled on the sides. Her hazel eyes, ready smile, and soft voice complemented her ability to multitask: she could answer phones while talking to patients in front of her and placating others. She never seemed to get flustered. She had the endearing ability to jump up and cradle your hand and call you *Hon*, and look into your eyes. This maneuver melted even the crankiest patients. Karl had chosen well.

I cleared my throat self-consciously.

"Anyone signed up to see me?"

"Not so far, Dr. Mathur. They're all here for Dr. Becker."

"Okay."

"But I have had some people call and ask about you. Maybe someone will call back and make an appointment."

"Let me know."

I went back to the coffee machine and slowly refilled, trying hard to look nonchalant. The laughter and talking was dying down. I surveyed the space, selected one of Karl's hunting magazines, and settled down. I glanced at pictures of victorious hunters kneeling next to large bucks, holding them up by their horns. *All it takes is patience,* one of them explained helpfully. I threw it down, disgusted.

A few minutes later, Amber got up and walked away from her desk to the restroom, about fifteen feet away. She closed the door and drew the bolt. A minute later, the air was rent by a rude sputtering, which stopped abruptly and started again as a bubbly screeching, its pitch rising and falling. It sounded like someone playing the trumpet while coughing.

I jumped to my feet, alarmed. The sound went on relentlessly, churning and vulgar, with gurgling and frothing and squirting sounds along with unmistakable strains. Everyone looked at the bathroom in astonishment. In the waiting room, the patients dropped their magazines and looked up; some stood up, in puzzlement and apprehension. The door opened hastily, and Amber bounded out, red with embarrassment.

"I *swear* that wasn't me! I *swear* it!"

Her flushed face and pained expression was too much for the staff. They burst into laughter and Amber ran to her seat and buried her head in her hands.

"I *swear* it! I heard it inside! It must be there!"

"It's Dr. Becker's new fart machine," Heather explained drily. "He thinks it's *funny*."

Dr. Becker came bursting out of a corner, his face convulsed and his body shaking with laughter.

"Dang it, Amber! Took me *forever* to get you! Thought you were *never* going to take a crap. You really fell for it!"

"Dr. Becker, that was so rude!"

"Hell, no! It was great! You should have seen the look on your face, Amber! Priceless!"

"Dr. Becker, you should be ashamed—"

"*Priceless!*"

"You should be ashamed! Ashamed of yourself! I was so scared! Shocked by that awful wailing!"

"Best damn catalog I ever had!" proclaimed Karl, wiping the tears from his eyes. "Guess I better go see my patients now. Ya'll watch out now! You hear! *All* of you!"

Karl retreated, chuckling, toward an examination room. The patient had come outside to see what all the commotion was about.

"What you doing? Get back inside!"

"What's all the commotion?"

"Made her jump right out her skin with that fart machine," he crowed. "Never seen her look like that. Dang!"

They disappeared into the examination room.

Heather looked up quietly.

"Dr. Becker takes some getting used to. When he did that to me the first time I cried and cried. But after that I loosened up. He just loves to see us flustered, so I just don't give him the pleasure. Just act as if nothing happened."

"How can you look like nothing happened," complained Amber, "When he just started a damn *tornado* under your . . .behind?"

"Just ignore him," advised Heather sagely. "Trust me, it's the only thing that works."

I finished my coffee and headed back down to the ER. I happened to go by the gift shop, run by volunteers, all elderly ladies in pink aprons.

"Welcome, Dr. Mathur," one sang out. "And how are you doing this fine morning?"

"Great, just great," I answered, looking around the small window-less nook nestled under the stairs.

There were flowers, an assortment of cards, books, soft toys, and a selection of toiletries. A bookrack displayed racy romances, with bare-chested men protecting busty women: *That Song of Desire, I Was Desperate for Love, Taming the Lion in Him, Queen of Temptation*, and *Passion in the Everglades* offered themselves up breathlessly. Several get-well cards lay open. There was a discreet notice from the funeral home. The local paper was prominently displayed near the cash register and warned of drought. The air smelt pleasantly of perfume and air freshener. I looked carefully at the lady who had addressed me.

"I'm Helga Geisinger, Doctor," she said, offering her hand. "I'm one of the volunteers."

She was a short, slender lady with tight skin and perfect makeup. Her lips were silky red and sharply defined. Her brown hair was deposited in tight curls about her head, and diamond earrings stuck out jauntily. She arched her eyebrows and regarded me with frank interest.

"You're married, but you don't wear a ring," she observed.

I noticed several rings on her hand as I shook it warmly. I wondered if *I* had such sharp powers of observation.

"Yes, you're right. I stopped wearing it in London after a year of wearing it because I was always taking it off to wash my hands and soap and dirt would accumulate, no matter what. So I decided that it would be better not to have it on."

"And your wife is okay with that, Doctor?"

"I think so. I hope so!"

"I live on the hill as well. I am your neighbor, just five houses down from you on the other side of the road. You know that great big oak tree that was hit by lightning?"

"Yes, of course."

"The house next to it is mine. Come by sometime, we'll have coffee. And bring that pretty wife of yours."

"Thank you, Mrs. Geisinger."

"Helga, Helga, please call me Helga. I'm not *that* old, honey!"

I walked into the ER, and the nurse, Gideon, sidled up and whispered to me.

"Were you talking to Helga Geisinger?"

"Yes."

"Did you know about her son?"

"No. What happened to him?"

"Nothing happened. But he's *gay!*"

I realized by his expression that he disapproved.

"Uh-uh. Gay, eh?"

"Yeah, *gay*. Lives with a *man*. Both of them, they're in the hair-salon business, in Florida. Shampoo, face creams, lip stuff. Made a *boatload* of cash. Guess they don't care about *that* kind of thing in Florida."

I was irritated again. I made an effort to stay calm. I debated whether to say something sharp like *we have several friends who are gay and we have had them over for dinner and it angers me when some idiot trashes them.* Would that be too much? What if I said, *how can you say anything so bigoted?*

But I didn't have to say anything. Gideon read my face and retreated.

"You still short on patients in the clinic?"

I flinched.

"What about the patient from Lancaster's?"

"The ambulance just picked him up. Should be here soon. You'd best hang around."

He glanced away.

"Doc, don't tell Miss Helga I told you about her son. Bless her heart!"

I sat down and looked around. I had spent a lot of weekends and evenings here. I surveyed the large yellow cardiac resuscitation cart, two tilting IV poles on wheels, and the floor lamp on a tripod. I gazed at the new boxes of surgical equipment: various sizes of needles, silk, nylon and catgut, IV tubing, cut-down kits, chest tubes, central line kits, and intubating sets. A small locked glass cupboard had ampoules and boxes of adrenaline, Benadryl, steroids, and other essential medicine. Everything had been reorganized neatly with precise typed labels. A handwritten label warned: DO NOT COVER NEEDLES and YOU MUST SIGN OUT FOR NARCOTICS, and THE RATTLESNAKE SERUM IS IN THE LITTLE FRIDGE. We had everything needed to keep you alive, I mused, till we could get you to a *real* hospital.

There was a clamor in the corridor, and the door burst open. A couple of paramedics rushed in, pulling in a stretcher.

"Thank God you're here, Doc," Carlos, the leader, shouted. "He's cut *real bad!*"

He was indeed. He was in his mid-twenties, but looked even younger. He was a pale, gaunt man, half-sitting up on the stretcher, with stringy red hair and marmalade stubble. He was looking raptly at his right forearm which he held up rigidly with his left and cried, *"Git it out! Git it out!"* His right forearm was shrouded in a blood-spattered towel. Gideon snatched it off.

I gasped. The right forearm had been pierced just above the wrist by a long jagged shaft of wood, and the wedge protruded out from the back of the forearm halfway up. There were many bruises, scratches, and abrasions on the hand and forearm as well as a few deep lacerations near the point of entry.

"Doc, this here's Colton Connally Huckabee! Works at Lancaster Manufacturing! Wood shredder backed up on him!"

We forced him to lie down flat and started an IV on the other arm. He wailed and turned over, twisting to keep the right side aloft, not allowing the wood to touch any surface. I scanned his fact-sheet. No medications, no allergies, no past surgeries.

"Demerol! Let's give him some Demerol!" I ordered. "Fifty mg, stat. Pour in the fluids, D5 saline, wide open. And let's give him some Unasyn, three grams, now. Double-check his allergies first!"

I tried to get some information, but he was in agony and answered in moans and grunts. Most of the history came from Carlos.

"One of the shredders jus' backed up. Started shootin' out the wood 'stead a' shreddin' it. Jes happened so quick. A big piece jes shot out and got 'im! Poor guy, din' know what hit 'im." Carlos explained. "Colton Huckabee's his name. Jes call 'im Colt."

"Any allergies?" I asked.

"Nope."

Colton cried out in pain. We eased him down again and quickly cut off his shirt. I called for an X-ray and administered the Demerol. I looked carefully at the piece of wood. It was half an inch wide in places and tapered at both ends.

"It's *killin'* me! Git it *out!*"

His mother and wife burst into the room, and his wife almost fainted. His wife was as tall and as lean; she was blonde and wore a short blue apron that said *Hotspur Supermarket*. His mother was in a dressing

143

gown, her red hair trailing like a pennant. His wife kissed his face as he writhed and his mother cried. I had them escorted out politely, but they kept coming back. Once the Demerol had its effect, I put a clean towel under the limb and rested it down carefully. I cleaned the entire right upper limb with iodine from the shoulder downward, and then cleaned it again with alcohol. I noticed that a lot of the bleeding was coming from minor abrasions that did not need any further treatment. I carefully checked the two main arteries in the forearm, the radial on the thumb side and the ulnar on the other, and found them to be pulsating strongly. That was a good sign, meaning that they had not been damaged.

"His arteries okay, Doc?" Carlos asked.

"Yes," I responded. "Fortunately for Colton, the two main arteries run down the sides of the forearm and he's been punctured in the middle, in between the two major vessels. That's good for him."

That reassured his wife and mother. I did a quick general exam, listening to his heart and lungs and abdomen and then palpated his abdomen. He was able to move all other muscle groups and sensation was intact everywhere else. I ordered a tetanus shot because Colton was unsure of his vaccinations.

"I'm going to call the ICU in Abilene," I announced. "We've got to get him to an orthopedic specialist."

Colton started to stir and moan.

"Hurtin'. . . I'm *hurtin' bad, Doc, hurtin' bad.*"

"Doc, he's *hurtin'*," Carlos explained, helpfully.

I looked up.

"Repeat the Demerol. Fifty mg, IV. How are his vitals?"

"Stable, Doc," Gideon responded.

"Watch the blood pressure. He's lost a lot of blood and Demerol can drop his blood pressure, okay?"

"Systolic is ninety, Doc!" Gideon said.

"Not good enough! Run that bag wide open!"

"You got it!"

We obtained X-rays of the arm and forearm. No fractures. The wood cast a wicked gray shadow obliquely in between the two bones of the forearm, the radius and the ulna. No metal fragments. I double-checked, and Joe watched grimly. I was able to get the orthopedic surgeon on call in Abilene, and told him the story.

"Well, if he's stable, why don't you just pull the wood out?" the surgeon asked.

"I don't feel comfortable doing that. I mean, I've never done that. How would I do that? And what if there was more bleeding?"

"Well, you just said his arteries were good. Were they or weren't they?"

"They were good."

"And it's in the center, so go ahead. Yank it out, then get another X-ray. Then call me back. You can do it."

He hung up. I turned with some trepidation to the staff. I was a gastroenterologist, trained in internal medicine, gastroenterology, liver disease, liver transplantation and, most recently, in the measurement of DNA in colon cancer cells. Yanking jagged wood out of a forearm? Why not?

"He says we should take it out. Do we have anything to pull it out?"

"I've got a big electrical pliers in the ambulance, Doc! That sucker'll grab the wood!" Carlos offered.

"Great! Go get it. And give me lots of lidocaine. Two percent with epi. About fifty cc."

I loaded up a twenty-cc syringe with lidocaine and attached a fine, long twenty-two-gauge needle. Carefully, I injected all around the entry wound, going deeper and deeper as I deadened successive layers. I pulled back on the syringe repeatedly to make sure there was no return of fluid or blood. Gideon lifted up the forearm and I contorted beneath it and resumed the same process on the other side, going deeper and deeper.

Carlos returned with a pair of giant pliers, and held them up for all to see. He opened and closed it, displayed the width of its jaws, and then offered it to me for final approval. I looked at Colton; he was listless and drowsy. He was also sweating profusely. I took a deep breath and decided to go ahead with the removal. We wiped down the pliers with alcohol and I put on sterile surgical gloves. Carlos and his junior, Chase, held the forearm rigidly, one at the elbow, the other at the wrist.

"Go for it, Doc!" they chorused.

There was more wood sticking out on the palmar side than the other, so I grabbed the free end of the wood from that side. I pulled gently.

Nothing.

I pulled a little more.

No movement.

I twisted gently from side to side. Nothing.

"Doc, he's waking up. You want to give him more Demerol?" Carlos asked.

I ignored Carlos and twisted harder. The wood remained embedded, as though set in cement. I imagined the blood and the macerated tissues inside the forearm, clotted and locked in at the jagged edges. The more I waited, the harder it would set. I grasped the pliers with both hands and pulled harder.

"Attaboy, Doc!" Chase grunted.

Colton was waking up and I saw the paramedics struggling. I had to do something more forceful. I raised one leg and jammed it against the pedestal. I moved one hand near the jaws and wrenched mightily, grasping the base of the wood and using my entire weight to pull back, keeping my net force in the same straight line as the wood. There was a sickening squelch and the shard moved out an inch. His mother gasped and covered her mouth. There was a burst of blood from both sides of the forearm and Colton screamed.

"Mudda-fugga! *Mudda-fugga! Fuggin muddafugga!*"

"I'm sorry, Colton! I'm trying to get it out of you!"

I stopped, and saw that the wood was no longer protruding from the other side of the forearm. I waited for Colton to calm down and resumed my efforts. With the same force in the same direction, I pulled and twisted and paused, pulled and paused, imagining the adherent coagulated muscle peeling off the wood like Velcro. A crater appeared at the point of entry, and more dark blood and fluid streamed out. His mother and wife cried out and Gideon lunged forward with gauze and applied pressure. The process gradually became slightly easier, and I kept up steady pressure. There was a final *pop* and I had the entire mass out.

I lifted the piece of wood up in awe. It looked like a bayonet. There were gasps all around.

"*Gawd damn* freakin' . . . sorry, Doc. Got carried away," Gideon said.

We repeated the X-ray. Everything looked good. I called the orthopedic surgeon back. He sounded pleased.

"Good job! How come we never heard of you before? Where are you from?"

"Actually, I'm from Houston. I trained in internal medicine and gastroenterology. I'm here to get my green card."

"Helluva job, gastro man! Send Colton my way, set up an early appointment, I'll check him out tomorrow or whenever. Be sure to send him out on some antibiotics."

"I was going to send him out on Keflex or Augmentin," I answered.

"Sounds good, gastro man. Dress the wound, no stitches, of course. Send him my way. Thanks!" he said and signed off.

We decided to keep Colton there for observation. I went back upstairs, drained. As I entered, Amber turned around and looked at me with a smile.

"Dr. Mathur, you have a patient waiting to see you. She's been waiting forty minutes. Can I have Tamara put her in a room now? Tamara's covering for Sharon."

The news went through me like an electric shock.

I have a new patient! She waited to see me! Excellent!

A phantom of doubt crossed before my mind. *Am I ready? What if she asks a question that I know nothing about?* I suppressed those thoughts and forced a wan smile. Again, I did my best to appear nonchalant.

"Excellent. Who is it?"

"Mrs. Thelma Trotter. She's from Cold Creek."

Cold Creek was a small community about fifteen miles away, noted for its pecan orchards and its annual dove hunt and cook-off.

"And her sister's with her too. Name's Velma."

"Thelma and Velma," I repeated.

I would try to greet them by name.

"Tell Tamara to put them in room one, I'll be right there."

"Well, room one is taken. Dr. Becker already has a patient there."

"Well, okay. What about room two? Or three?"

"I think he has patients waiting in all of them. Wait, I'll ask Tamara."

Tamara was an LVN, a licensed vocational nurse. She was in her midforties but looked a great deal older. She had smoked heavily as a teenager and in her twenties, and it had hardened her face. Her bright brown eyes still twinkled in a leathery face, drawn thin and etched with sharp furrows as if by an artist who had forgotten to erase all the mistakes. She was extremely proud of her buoyant blonde hair, which fell in extravagant cascades around her slender shoulders.

"You'll have to wait. Dr. Becker is talking to someone in three, and he has patients waiting in one and two. But you won't have to wait long. He *doesn't-take-too-much-time*."

Tamara raised her eyebrows, rolled her eyes and handed me the chart.

"No, he *never-takes-too-much-time*, our Dr. Becker, if you get what I mean," Tamara said.

I avoided her gaze. I didn't want to say or even imply anything about Dr. Becker. After all, he had been good to me. He had shown me around the hospital, shown me how to remove fish hooks, apply a plaster of Paris cast, how to use Chinese finger splints, and how to cut a cast open. I didn't want to get drawn into office politics and jeopardize everything. I knew that everything I said would find its way to his ears. *Let it go, let it go.*

"The ER needs you, Dr. Mathur. Your patient Colton is complaining of pain. They want you to come down."

I glanced at Tamara.

"Put the patient and her sister in the first room that becomes available. Tell them I'll be right back. And . . . "

"And tell Dr. Becker not to see her?"

I looked up in astonishment. *Is everything in life this obvious?*

"Yeah, I'll tell Dr. Becker to keep his snout outta your trough. No problem," Tamara said.

I got up and walked down briskly. I couldn't decide whether I liked or disliked Tamara. If she could be so sharp about Dr. Becker, she could be equally stinging in her remarks about me. However, she was clearly not a fan of Dr. Becker, and that could be helpful. I swept past the lab and the volunteers shop at the bottom of the stairs and slipped back into the ER. Gideon handed me the clipboard.

"He's still hurting a lot, Doc. Says there's got to be another piece or two."

Colton was writhing back and forth, holding has battered forearm aloft like a lioting oail.

"Hurting real bad, real firkin bad, Doc!"

I examined his forearm again. The whole forearm was swollen like a sausage. The tissues were bloated and glistening with sweat, iodine, and alcohol. I tenderly poked the large wound in the center with my gloved finger.

"Jesus Chrise!" he yelled, "*Chrise!* That's ferkin' painful, dammit!"

His mother apologized. I shrugged.

I turned the forearm around. On both sides, the skin flaps looked bruised and irregular but the tissue felt soft. I couldn't feel any other pieces of wood. I looked again at the X-ray, but wood is not completely radio-opaque like bone or metal. I didn't see anything suspicious.

"Okay, let's give him another twenty-five of Demerol IV, now. I'm going to look and feel all over the forearm."

"Just twenty-five? Doc, he's had over two hundred and it's not holding him!" Gideon pointed out.

"Okay, give him fifty. But slow IV, don't push it. Take your time, five minutes. And check his blood pressure again."

"Pressure's fine, Doc. Already checked it. You told me last time."

Once Colton had calmed down, I examined the forearm again. He winced as I felt laterally around the main wound. Nothing. I took off the glove, cleaned my hand and fingers with alcohol, and palpated gingerly with a bare fingertip.

Still nothing.

I suspected that there *was* a splinter still there. The swelling obscured the clue I was looking for, the telltale bump of a splinter's tail. I went over the area back and forth with my bare fingertips. Nothing. *I am missing something.* The machine must have shot out more than just one missile. Some smaller pieces must have been ejected, like birdshot. There *must* be at least one more sliver of wood, maybe two, following roughly the same trajectory but diverging slightly, I reasoned. But the swelling obscured everything. A sudden thought struck me.

"Let's raise his hand up! Let's use the Chinese finger traps to hold his four fingers and lift up his forearm as high as possible, and try to reduce the swelling. Then I'll look again."

We raised his forearm up gently and slid his four fingers into the finger traps. These look like the individual fingers cut off a glove, but made of wire mesh. Wires from the tips of the four traps suspended them from a horizontal metal rod, making them look like the four fingers of a hand reaching up to a flat line. We eased Colton's fingers into the four traps, and the tissue bulging in between the mesh prevented them from slipping out. The arrangement gripped his fingers firmly and allowed us to elevate the limb. We raised his forearm up vertically and waited. I called Tamara in the clinic.

"Mrs. Trotter understands," Tamara said. "She says, if it was her in the ER, she'd a wanted you to see her first. But she says she has to leave by three forty-five, she has a beauty appointment."

"A *beauty appointment?*"

"She got a appointment at Mitsy's beauty shop. Wednesday at four, she's got to be there. Get her hair done an all. Hair's big deal in Texas, Doc, 'specially for little old ladies."

"She's going to miss a clinic appointment for a visit to the *beauty shop?*"

"Happens all the time, Doc. Don't sweat it. Do what you got to do. She can reschedule for tomorrow."

Upset, I returned grudgingly to my challenge. Ten agonizing minutes had passed. I waited another five. I thought about calling home, but decided against it. Everyone could hear me. I glanced back at the patient. A scruffy little redheaded boy had appeared at his side. He wore dirty jeans, no shirt, and no shoes. He gazed at his dad with his mouth open and, when he saw the bloody forearm pulled up in the Chinese finger-trap apparatus, a thrill went through his body.

"Hoo-wee!" he cried, twisting with excitement. "Thass a real *sugga-mugga!*"

There was a shocked silence. Then everyone spoke at once.

"What!"

"What you say?"

"*Junior!*"

"Junior! Ah can't *believe* you jes said thet!"

Junior withdrew a few steps, then pulled himself up.

"Dad says that all the time!"

Fifteen minutes after elevating his forearm, I donned a fresh pair of surgical gloves and painted the forearm and the gloves with plenty of alcohol. I used my fingertips to glide up and down the forearm, like shaving with and against the grain. I thought I felt something but it was too vague. I repeated it but the result was still the same. In desperation, I ripped off the gloves. I washed my hands twice and sprayed them with alcohol, and then ran my bare fingertips down.

Then, *something!* Yes, something! It was about half an inch to the right and slightly above the main wound, in the area I suspected. *It's all a matter of probability,* I thought. *Got to look in the area of maximum probability.* I slipped on magnifying glasses and confirmed my discovery. What seemed sharp was a brown stub, just barely visible above a faded iodine veldt. I grasped the end firmly with a fine-tipped forceps, taking care not to break it. I pulled back, holding my breath. Like a conjuror's trick, a two-inch sliver slithered out and then stopped, tenting the skin. I tugged again, and the skin rose in response. There was an edge that was catching, like a ledge. The nurses recoiled.

"Don' break it, Doc! You'll never get it out then!"

But I was tired of being patient. I wanted to go up and see my patient. So I tugged again. It snapped with a pop. I grabbed the tented skin before it collapsed. The broken upper part was at the end of my forceps.

"Quick, get me some lidocaine, two percent, with epi. Just three or four cc. And give me a small scalpel blade now!"

Colton stirred. The phone rang and he woke up, looking dazed. I lunged for the scalpel packet, ripped it open and used my left hand to hold the splinter remnant close to the skin. I pulled it in the same direction, tented the skin some more, and swiftly made a small incision, an eighth of an inch, to open the passage. Colton yelped. A bead of watery blood welled up immediately. I jabbed into the wound with the tip of my forceps and grasped the remnant. I tugged again and again, like a dog fighting over a bone. I had to grasp the fragment before it disappeared into the depths.

There was a sound like a bubble popping and another inch of black wood burst out. The tented skin collapsed. I lifted the sliver clear and inspected the tiny notch. I triumphantly displayed it to everyone in the room, like a trophy. Carlos and Chase looked awestruck. Gideon was unimpressed.

"Will someone answer the damn phone? He's finally got it out, now!"

Carlos picked up the phone. I cleaned the site and checked it one last time. I released the finger splints and lowered his forearm. Gideon applied a clean bandage.

"It's your nurse, Doc," Carlos said," She says your patient is asking how much longer."

"Tell her I'll be right there!"

I washed quickly. As I left, his mother came up.

"God bless you, Doctor. God bless you an' yo family."

She squeezed my forearm and returned to her son and grandson. Colt's wife massaged the sides of his head and his mother scooped up the boy and crooned and rocked him. Gideon came up to me, always keen to have the last word.

"May *God bless you*, Doc," he said, mimicking the accent and handing me the clipboard to finish the paperwork. "I hope He does, too, Doc, because that's all that *you're* going to get. They have no insurance. They have no money. They're poor as church mice. *You* won't get a dime! All yo fine fine work's fo Jesus!"

As I bounded up the stairs, I wondered if I remembered everything I was supposed to know. *What if the Trotters asked something I had forgotten? What if she had a rare disease and I could not even begin to tell her anything meaningful? What if she walked out on me, disgusted? What if she had already walked out?*

I burst in to the clinic and checked myself. I walked as calmly as I could through the office and toward the examination rooms. I picked up my clipboard and asked Tamara as nonchalantly as possible, "So where is she?"

Tamara looked up. She was sporting a half-smile.

"Room three. Got to warn you, Dr. Becker is in there!"

"*What!*" I burst out, and scrambled.

Just as I reached the door, it swung open and Karl came out with a curious expression on his face. He thrust the patient file at me, announced, "She's all yours, buddy!" and stomped down the corridor.

I felt a pang of relief and gratitude. *I still had a patient! A new patient from out of town! I needed to get patients from the little hamlets around Hotspur! I knew Mrs. Trotter wrote a column in the local paper, so she would know a lot of people and might recommend me!* It seemed so important. I wanted to remember every detail.

I took a deep breath, knocked, and entered. The examination room was large and empty. A generous window framed a step-down transformer but let in plenty of natural light. To the right of the window was a small bathroom, the door ajar. A small Norman Rockwell print graced one wall, the other had an eye chart. There were two women sitting stiffly side by side and there was a metal stool next to them. I sat down on the stool and maneuvered into position, facing them. They were in their seventies, with keen faces and similar features. Layers of makeup frosted their faces and intelligent black eyes gleamed back at me. I paused to take in their hair, which was scalloped in stiff white curls tinted with blue, their exuberance disciplined by strict cotton scarves. Two large handbags perched on their knees, buttressed by nodular fingers, created a wall.

"Good afternoon! Thanks for waiting. I was tied up in the ER and I . . ."

"Oh, you don't have to worry. That was Michelle's boy down there. I used to teach Colton in Sunday school. If it was me there, I'd a-wanted you there myself."

"This here's Velma, and I'm Thelma Trotter. We're sisters. Hope you don't mind both of us being here."

"Not at all. Actually, I encourage it. It always helps to have two pairs of eyes and ears in the room, rather than one."

The two sisters exchanged glances and nodded.

"Well, Miss Velma, how are you doing today? How can I help you?"

"I'm having problems with my blood pressure," she explained, leaning forward over her purse, "and I've been trying so hard to get it under control!"

"Sister, *Dr. Becker* has been trying to get it under control."

"Yes, I mean, Dr. Becker has been trying. Bless his heart, he's a good man, and I love his wife and his kids and he's a God-fearing man, but I guess I just need some help. I hated having to walk past him and come to you."

They exchanged glances.

"Sister, you are going to have a *stroke!* Just like Mamma did! Is that what you want?"

"What kind of blood pressure readings are we talking about?"

"Real high, Doc. Sometimes it's normal, below one hundred thirty on the upper number but it gets to one hundred and seventy and one hundred and eighty a lot of the time. And when it gets that way I can tell. I feel dizzy and tired. Just not right. Mostly in the evenings."

"Have you had any chest pains or shortness of breath?"

"No. But once I felt short of breath after I had been watching TV at night, then I coughed and coughed, but I think that was bronchitis."

"Have you had any problems with your eyes or your kidneys?"

"Well, I have macular degeneration and I do get urinary infections sometimes."

"Do you know if you have any weakness of your kidneys?"

"What do you mean?"

"Well, have you had any blood tests that showed that you had weak kidneys?"

"Haven't had a blood test in a long time. Maybe a year."

"Okay, well, we can get that. It would be useful to check your kidney functions. We can check something called the creatinine level, a blood test that gives us an idea of the kidney function. Also, we should check your potassium level. Any other medical concerns?"

"Not that I can think of right now."

"Are you careful about your salt and water intake?"

"Oh, yes. Real careful. No added salt, no salty foods."

"You take any decongestants? Allergy medicines?"

"Allergy medicines? Like Benadryl and all? Why?"

"Decongestants can raise your blood pressure."

"No. No allergy medicines."

I examined her carefully, using a format I had honed. I went over her radial and pedal pulses, palpated her neck and armpits for lymph nodes and checked for swollen veins. I listened to her heart and lungs, then her abdomen. I examined her abdomen and then sat her up. I flashed a light in her mouth and then in her eyes, checking for the reflexive changes in the pupils. I checked for sensation and coordination and finally used a knee hammer to check her reflexes. She was cooperative, and seemed pleased and surprised when her legs jerked. Both sisters chuckled.

"Haven't had that checked in a long time, sister!"

I reviewed her medications.

"I see you're on a pretty high dose of ACE inhibitors. You're taking a hundred and fifty mg of captopril. That's high. You're also taking a beta-blocker, atenolol, at a hundred mg daily. While those are definitely very good, very safe medicines, they are not doing the job for you. We have to get your blood pressure down."

"What should I do?"

"I recommend we change the captopril to a different kind of medicine called a calcium channel blocker, maybe something called amlodipine."

"It's not going to be dangerous?"

"Would you put your mother on it?" Thelma questioned.

"I *have* my mother on it," I countered, truthfully. I thought of my mother, briefly, in India, and recalled that she was pleased with my choice of an inexpensive and effective remedy for her hypertension.

"Well, is it safe if it blocks calcium? I have osteoporo-something. I think I need my calcium."

"This medicine won't aggravate your osteoporosis."

"That's it, that's it! Osteoporosis! Sister had a fracture of her back from osteo-that. Isn't that right, sister?"

"Surely," Thelma said. "Had to get shots in my back to fix it all. Still hurts a little."

"What are you taking for it?"

"Calcium, regular as clockwork."

"And what else?"

"That's it. What else do you need?"

"You need to take vitamin D along with your calcium and you should take another medicine to help the calcium stay in the bones."

"Sister takes Caltrate plus D twice daily," interjected Thelma, helpfully.

"Then the vitamin D is taken care of, but she still needs to take something to stop the osteoporosis. You can think of calcium and vitamin D like bricks, but you still need cement to make the bricks stick together. You need both bricks and cement to make a wall, you can't build a strong wall with just the one and not the other. Medicines like Fosamax are the cement that help hold the calcium in the bones together."

They smiled in understanding.

"I like that," Velma said. "Bricks and cement. Makes sense."

"Daddy was a bricklayer," Thelma added.

They got stiffly to their feet, still holding their purses.

"Thank you, Doc. We—"

She broke off in mid-sentence. A high-pitched sound had started up. It was rapidly followed by sounds of straining, with paroxysms of blubbering and boiling, all building up to an obnoxious screech. The sound then burst like an exploding rocket and broke up into several smaller bubbling symphonies, which stretched on and on. I froze in horror, speechless. I tried to say something elegant and dismissive but I couldn't. The fart machine blared, and I floundered.

Thelma and Velma smiled patiently back at me.

I couldn't believe it.

My fledgling career in medicine was being interrupted by a fart machine.

"We *know* it's not *you*," said Velma sweetly.

Thelma giggled.

"It's Dr. Becker's fart machine. I think he hid it in your bathroom before you got here."

They turned and walked out, buffeted by a second roar of angrier intestinal spasms. I gathered up my notes and marched out after them, trying to maintain as much dignity as possible. Roars and blasts and tooting followed us, rising to a crescendo, and made the sisters shudder as they approached the checkout window. Amber's face was red with suppressed merriment, and she kept her quivering lips together with difficulty. Dr. Becker made no such effort. He burst into view, guffawing.

"Did I get you or what? I got you so bad!"

He was laughing so much that the rest of the office broke down. Even some patients in the waiting room picked up on it and smiled broadly or snickered. I tried not to smile and darted into the relative obscurity of a cubbyhole behind the checkout desk.

"So how was everything?" asked Amber, as she made a follow-up appointment.

There was a pause as the two sisters eyed each other and thought it over.

Then Velma turned back and declared, "I surely do like my little Mexican doctor!"

Another gale of laughter erupted and I couldn't hold back, either. I laughed out loud.

Karl boomed.

"Yeah, Sandy! Laugh at yourself! Let it go! Let it go!"

CHAPTER TWELVE

Sparky Goes Out

The pathology report said it all.

Metastatic small cell cancer. Primary could be lung or upper airway.

My mouth dried. I remembered Sparky Cummins, the man who had been admitted with pneumonia. I had been worried about him, and I had biopsied a small mass on his chest wall. The small lump was cancer, and what was worse, it was cancer that had spread from somewhere else. That made it an advanced cancer, stage four, the worst situation.

Must be a lung cancer, given his smoking. It must be in the lower airway, blocking a branch of the breathing tube called the bronchus. The obstruction is why he developed pneumonia and why there was scarring and why the trachea, the tube in the neck that splits into the bronchi, was pulled over to that side rather than pushed away. I had suspected this all along, and had seen it in Houston and London, but the shock of seeing the report made me pause.

I showed the report to my nurse, Tamara.

"Did we ever hear from Sparky Cummins again?"

"No, he didn't show up for his follow-up appointment."

"I'm not surprised. But he needs to come back now. His path report is bad."

"Cancer?"

"Yes, stage four."

"Jesus! You got to tell him!"

"I know he won't come in. I don't like to do this over the phone, but I have to talk to him personally, right away."

I steeled myself for the barrage of questions. *Are you sure? Could it be something else? Maybe just an infection? Can it be cured?*

Sparky did not pick up. He did not have a cell phone.

"You can call the police to go over to his house and check on him. Maybe he's just passed out or something."

"Why would he be passed out?"

Tamara shrugged and looked away.

"He drinks a lot. So does his wife. Everyone in town knows that."

"I suspected that, but wasn't sure."

"First they had their neighbor's son buy the booze. Even threw the empty bottles in someone else's trash. Then they stopped bothering. Just go and get it themselves now."

"Call the police, Tamara. Tell them to go check on the Cummins."

Tamara was quick. Within minutes, she had an update.

"They're on their way to the ER. Sparky says the pain is real bad."

The cancer was sitting on top of the rib and is now probably growing into it, burning into it like acid.

I went down and saw them in the ER. Sparky had lost at least fifteen pounds and looked withered. He spoke in short bursts. He was propping himself up with difficulty and holding his chest with his other hand. His wife, her face even more red, her hair still black, was even more shaky and crossed her arms to hide their trembling. She looked away.

"Hurts—right here, where you did—that thing."

"You mean, the biopsy?"

"Yeah, biopsy. Hurts—when ah—breathe deep."

His wife nodded.

"Hurts real bad. Real bad. Brings tears to his eyes!"

"Gotta breathe, real shallow like. Big breath's . . . what kills me!"

"Let me examine you."

I ordered the old chart and started the exam. Thinner, *not eating due to the pain and the painkillers, and the cancer itself.* Pale, *due to blood loss from coughing it up, but there could be other causes like ulcers from painkillers and anti-inflammatory medicines, and he's never had a colonoscopy so think about colon cancer as well.* His breasts were still large and seemed more prominent because of the weight loss. His breathing was rapid and shallow and he was sweating from the effort. Sparky leaned forward and supported himself with both arms. *Central bloating, swollen trunk with thin arms and legs, due to chronic steroid therapy and alcoholism.* There was exquisite tenderness around the mass under the breast that had doubled in size, turned purple, and looked like a fat leech. *It's definitely malignant, and the cancer is on the other side so it's a distant metastasis, not local extension, and that's stage four, the worst stage.* There were loud crackles in both lungs. I tapped with my fingers in the spaces between the ribs. Stony dullness, *a sign of fluid oozing from the cancer and filling up the chest cavity. It would compress the lungs and worsen the situation.*

I straightened up and cleared my throat. Sparky's wife, Esperanza, was sitting down. I sat down close to them.

"Actually, there's a lot to tell you. Sparky, I wanted to tell you and your wife about the results of the biopsy."

"Was it cancer?"

I paused and looked at them unblinkingly. *Should I say it? Should I?*

"Give it, straight!" he said.

I looked him in the eye.

"Yes. I'm sorry to say, it was cancer."

Sparky flinched. His wife burst into sobs. He looked down at the malignant mass on his chest. He looked up.

"So I got skin cancer?"

"Let me explain. The cancer cells on your biopsy are not skin cancer but cancer cells that started somewhere else."

Sparky shook his head and pulled back.

"No, no, no!"

"What does that mean, Sparky?" his wife asked.

"What he's—sayin is, it's cancer—from somewhere—else—spread t'skin."

He was still shaking his head in disbelief. His wife cupped her face with her hands in horror, speechless.

"Lung cancer!"

"Likely. Not sure, but likely."

Sparky looked away. He huffed for a minute, then spoke.

"I figured it was cancer. You did, too."

His wife shook her head.

"Always knew. Always knew—I'd die a'cancer. Knew it—minute—turned forty, bin smoking—since eight. Stole 'em, from Dad."

There was a short silence. His body quivered and his head drooped. His wife peered out the window and dabbed her eyes with a tissue. He looked up and blinked back tears. He spoke on the second attempt.

"So where—we go—from from here?"

"I can send you to a specialist in Abilene."

He shook his head.

"Heck no! No specialists—no goin'—Abilene—or anywhere!"

"It would be better and safer for you."

"What they—gonna do? No chemo—f'me! Ain't cutting—me!"

"Sparky, honey, maybe we should go."

"No!"

He shook his head and turned away.

"Doc, I . . . just gotta . . . get somethin'. . . fo' pain!"

"I'm going to take care of the pain, don't worry about that."

"We din come—see ya—no money!"

"Don't worry about it."

"Can't afford—high-priced—pain stickers."

"Them patches, Fenta something," his wife explained.

"Fentanyl patches. What about Darvocet or Tylenol with codeine?"

"Like candy. Don't do a bit a'good," his wife said.

I shrugged.

"Sparky, you look pretty rough. How about if I just admit you? That way we can get things under control, then let you go home when you're better."

He started shaking his head before I could finish.

"Don't—want."

"Sparky, honey, I can't take you home like this!"

"I *don't*—want!"

I put a hand on his shoulder.

"Sparky, give me just two days. I'll do what I can, then you can go home."

Sparky shook his head and looked away.

"Wise guy! You—fool me?"

"Just two days. That's all."

He turned to his wife.

"What you—think, Mama?"

"Do what the doctor tells you, Sparky honey!"

Sparky nodded.

"Okay. Two days. I want—same room!"

I was puzzled. Esperanza spoke quietly.

"He likes the view from one-oh eight. He can see Nueces Street."

I shrugged and requested the room.

I went to see Sparky in his hospital room later that day, before going home. He was sitting up in bed, leaning forward, with a facemask for oxygen, and a fan blowing straight at him. I could hear him wheeze. He lifted his mask to speak.

"Hey, Doc! I'm feeling . . . a lot better!"

"Glad to hear it!"

"Thanks for—the room!"

I listened to his lungs again. *Not much better.* There was little movement of air in his lungs.

"You've still got a long way to go! Your lungs don't sound too good!"

Sparky nodded and sucked more oxygen before talking.

"Doc, can I have some—more pain medicine? I'm still hurtin'."

"You're on morphine every two hours as needed."

"Just not enough."

"Okay, I'll double it. I'll go tell the nurses. You're getting antibiotics, by the way, and your breathing treatments should be every two hours."

I moved to the door.

"Thanks, Doc."

I paused as I left the room.

"Anything else?"

"What did the X-ray show?"

I had hoped to avoid discussing it. Sparky sensed it and sat up.

"Real bad, Doc?"

"Well, there are more shadows in the lungs."

"What's that mean?"

"There's infection or cancer spreading in the lungs."

"But I was on . . . some antibiotics when I . . . was home! How could it be . . . infected?"

"Sometimes bugs get resistant to antibiotics."

He shook his head and looked away.

"No, Doc. Ain't infection."

He looked out the window silently. He looked out onto oak-lined College Avenue, with a median, where it intersected Nueces. I noticed the cross there. A few cars and trucks were parked on both streets.

"How bad?"

"What do you mean?"

"You know what—I mean."

I walked back inside and sat down near him.

"The final report's not back from Abilene."

"But what do you . . . you think?"

I hesitated.

"I'm not a radiologist. Let's wait on the report. I don't want to tell you something until I'm sure."

"Doc, I trust you. Wouldn't be here . . . if I didn't."

He paused and breathed hard.

"What do—you think, Doc?"

I didn't know what to say. The X-ray looked terrible.

"It's not pretty. Lots of new shadows."

"Right side?"

"Both sides."

He winced.

"Ribs look okay?"

"No."

"Cancer eating my ribs?"

I hesitated.

"I think so."

His wife was watching me, speechless.

"So I don't have a . . . a chance, do I?"

"I don't know that. I think you should go to Abilene."

"And do what?"

"See a specialist! Maybe they could give you something, do something!"

He shook his head wearily.

"Thanks for everything, Doc!"

He waved me away.

"Go. Go home now."

I felt uneasy. I knew the situation was hopeless, but I was concerned. *Am I sitting on him, wasting time while he inched closer to death? Should I force him to go? Am I at risk of malpractice by keeping him here on comfort measures only? I had him sign a form, I think, but will that be enough? Dr. Bulent has the State Board sniffing around.*

I wondered if I had documented everything properly. I remembered being upset about my shirt and tie and pulling my tie out of the trash the first time I had seen him. I made a mental note to write something in the chart about his refusal to go to Abilene.

———

Priya and Anjali had been busy. Hand paintings adorned the living room and the girls pranced around in delight, explaining them, telling me over and over about splashing color on each other, smearing the paper, squeezing glitter glue and sticking feathers on their master-pieces. They made huge soap bubbles and chased each other with them. We had waffles for dinner, Anjali's favorite.

"I think you're going to have a hard time getting them to sleep, they're so excited!" Maya warned me.

She was right. After their baths, they lay gurgling and chattering in the dark. I turned out the light in the corridor and sat down at the threshold.

"Now calm down, both of you, and go to sleep."

"I don't want to sleep!" Priya declared.

"You know it's nine o'clock."

"I don't feel sleepy!" Priya shot back.

"Just wait."

"We watch TV?" Anjali asked, hopefully.

"No. Now calm down."

"Can you tell us a story?" Priya pleaded.

"Do you want to hear a story about Akbar and Birbal?"

"Okay!" they chorused.

"You want to hear the one where Birbal pretended to be a poor man looking for somewhere to stay?"

"And Akbar says, to go find a cheap hotel?"

"Yes, that one."

"No. That's too sad. Birbal says we all die and so we all live in hotels."

"That's the whole story right there!"

"No, no, too sad. Tell us the one about the poo!"

"Again?"

"Poo one!" Anjali chortled.

I resigned myself to the poo story. My grandmother would not have approved, but it always made them laugh. They were finally satisfied. I sat on the floor in the darkness and waited for them to fall asleep.

"Best day *ever!*" Anjali whooped.

———

The next morning I went to see Sparky. He had several family members in the room. The men wore crisp white shirts and jeans and walked stiffly, and the women wore dark skirts and jackets and bustled around offering cookies and coffee. A few young children in formal clothes buzzed around and were scooped up and anchored by their parents and told to hush. The room smelt of tobacco and perfume. I introduced myself and shook hands with all of them. They thanked me, then hugged and kissed Sparky and his wife, and retreated to the corridor. I closed the door and examined Sparky. He was still wheezing and his lungs were severely congested. A little more air was getting in, and he looked less tired. His speech had improved.

"I'm trying to avoid too much . . . too much dope, Doc!"

"You don't have to do that!"

"I know. I wanted to speak. To my family."

"I know you signed a form saying you did not want us to put a breathing tube into your lungs."

"Yeah," he said, flatly, looking out the window toward Nueces Street.

"You still sure about that?"

"Yeah."

I looked around and nodded at his wife. *I have a witness.*

"So if your breathing gets worse, you don't want us to put a tube in and hook you up to a ventilator?"

"No!"

"You can change your mind anytime."

He shook his head and dismissed me.

His wife flagged me down in the corridor.

"He's gonna need something for nerves."

"I know."

"He drinks heavy. Real heavy."

"I know. I have him on thiamine and Librax, in case he has withdrawal."

She nodded, satisfied.

"He gonna talk to his lawyer 'bout his will."

"Okay. You know, he is really sick!"

"Oh, I know. He knows it."

"You know he may not make it."

"Yes."

She wiped her eyes and looked away.

"I wanna say thanks for putting up with him. He's hardheaded, he is."

"No problem."

"His lawyer's Teegarten."

"Teegarten? The DA?"

"Yeah. He's kin to us."

I thought back to my first weekend on call in Hotspur. I had looked after a young man who had a severe reaction to a bee sting. His uncle, the DA, had not been confident about me and had been calling Karl for help. I was a little concerned. The young man had survived, so I reassured myself. *Nothing to worry about.*

―――――――――

I dropped in again at four thirty that afternoon. Sparky was sitting up in bed, washed and brushed, his hair slicked back and his ruddy face glowing. He finished a breathing treatment and waved me to a chair. The room was cool and a table fan was blowing on his face. He spoke more calmly.

"Honey, my mouth's dry. Coffee?"

His wife nodded.

"Want some, Doc?"

"No thanks."

"He's goin' home. He's . . . coffee with the missus," Sparky said.

He turned to me conspiratorially.

"Heard your missus, real good lookin'!"

I smiled.

"Lucky dawg, you!"

He straightened and looked out the window. He labored to breathe for a few minutes, then spoke looking forward.

"Thanks for putting up with me."

"No problem."

"I shoot my mouth."

"Many people do."

"That morphine, that's good stuff!"

"Yes, it is. You don't need to suffer."

"Yeah, yeah."

165

"Are you getting enough pain medicine? Enough to deal with, you know, the suffering? I don't want you to suffer."

There was a long pause. He looked out the window and opened and closed his mouth, then closed his eyes and bowed.

"Suffering. *Suffering*."

He shook his head and wiped his eyes.

"Doc, I want to tell you something."

His wife came back and handed him his coffee. He took a few sips and placed it down near the fan. She sat on the side of the bed.

"I want to tell you about our suffering."

He squeezed his wife's hand.

"This pain's nothin'. I'll tell you about *real* sufferin'."

His wife stood up, alarmed.

"I want to tell you 'bout our son."

"No!" she cried out.

"I *want* to tell you 'bout our son."

His wife stood up and cupped her hands awkwardly over his oxygen mask.

"No, don't say a thing! *Hush!*"

He shook his head and removed her hands.

"I *want* to tell you, tell you 'bout our son. Our eighteen-year-old son, Travis. Our eighteen-year-old son, who fell out the back, back of a pickup. Five years ago, on Nueces Street, couple blocks from here. I can see it, from here. I can see his cross."

That's why he wanted one-oh-eight.

His wife rubbed his forearm and swayed a little. I looked out and saw the white cross curbside midway on Nueces. I had noticed it the week we arrived.

"Our son just fell, just fell, fell out a pickup. Hit *hard*. Rushed 'im to Abilene. Helicopter an all. Died a' head injuries. Never woke up."

He looked at the window. His wife looked away.

"I'm so sorry to hear that!"

"I died with him, Doc. I bin sufferin', his mamma bin sufferin', somethin' fierce. I miss him, Doc! I miss him *every minute!*"

I didn't know what to say. He looked at me. His face was contorted, and his eyes were wide and fixed.

"Doc, I gotta ask you, you got kids?"

"Yes."

"Then, you can understand. He was my *little boy.*"

I looked away.

"He was eighteen, but he was my *little boy.* Straight-A student. Never a complaint bout 'im. Everbody loved 'im, girls specially. Good lookin' rascal he was, good lookin'. Sweet an' kind an' gentle, Doc, he was."

He shook his head and wiped his eyes with the blanket.

"He was everything, everything, *everything* I had, Doc. He was—*my joy, Doc, my sweet little boy*!"

My eyes burned and my throat closed up. I tried to hold it all back. He broke into sobs. Sparky and his wife hugged each other and cried together. I tried not to think of my own children.

"Why? *Why?* I can't make no sense of it."

I looked away and rubbed my eyes. It wouldn't look professional to tear up. I choked but said nothing. I didn't want to distract him, and I couldn't say anything that would help.

"Parent's nightmare, *worst* nightmare, *worst...*"

My throat tightened further and my eyes streamed.

"*Lost* my faith. Couldn't make no sense of it."

"Hush now! You've said enough!" Esperanza said.

"I loss faith, Doc! Now I wish I had faith!"

I stared back at him.

"But I can't! I can't! *Why him?*"

"Hush now! Now you gonna blaspheme!" his wife said.

"No, I ain't. I'm trying to come to peace with, with *whatever.*"

"Don't blaspheme!"

"No, Mama, I ain't gonna blaspheme."

"Good!"

We sat in silence. I watched Sparky's breathing settle down to an easier pace, and the sound of the fan was heard again. His wife walked to the window.

"You lookin' at Nueces Street?" Sparky said to his wife. "I can see it, see it from here."

She shuddered and kept her back to us.

Sparky looked at her standing in front of the window.

"I just don't understand. Why my little boy? Why *my* little boy? He was a good boy. Guess I could ask when I get there. But you know, I don' even know where I'm goin', and if there's even anythin' to go to!"

He slumped.

"So what's the answer, Doc? You got any ideas? What's the answer?"

The nurse came in with a tray.

"Morphine?"

Sparky looked at me and winked.

He held out his forearm with the IV port.

"Bring it on!"

═══════════════

They called me later that night.

"Doc, sorry to disturb you. Just wanted you to know that Mr. Cummins passed."

I thought back to the afternoon, to the ER and the previous visit.

Could I have done something differently?

"Was he comfortable?"

"Yes. He had just had some morphine."

"How did his wife take it?"

"Not well. She's gone. Doc, I think she's drinking again."

"Maybe. Thanks for letting me know."

Could I have done something differently? Could I have saved him?

I tossed and turned. I remembered the white floral cross with buntings fluttering on the side of Nueces Street. I imagined his son on that street, and the accident. I slept, sad and confused.

CHAPTER THIRTEEN

You Say You Want an Evolution

It was a Saturday morning and Maya was making pancakes for the girls. The warm air in the kitchen held the comforting smell of caramel and maple syrup and cooked fruit. The girls were jockeying for position at the table, to be close to the pancakes and have a good view of the TV. Everyone was still dressed in their pajamas and looking their morning worst when the doorbell rang. We froze.

"At this time?" Maya said.

"Who is it, Dad?" Priya asked, energized.

"Who, *who*, Dad?" Anjali said, after a pause. I wondered again about her hearing.

"Better put on a dressing gown. It might be a neighbor," said Maya .

I scurried off and reappeared in an old blue bathrobe. The doorbell rang again.

"Dad looks like a *magician!*" Priya observed.

"Don't you have anything better?" Maya remarked.

"Can't find it now. They seem to be in a hurry, don't they?"

I opened the door. A short, stout man in overalls waited there. He immediately grabbed my hand and shook it enthusiastically.

"How d'ye do? Dr. Mathur, I'm Mark Hastings."

He paused for effect. I felt I should be impressed. I paused and then invited him inside.

"Yes, of course. Mr. Hastings, come on in. We were just sitting down for breakfast."

"Sorry to interrupt you. Mornin', ma'am! Hello, kids!"

He walked straight into the kitchen and stood there, surveying the crew.

Priya and Anjali had long hair, strewn all over their faces, stuck down in places with dried syrup. Their faces were unwashed and their clothes stained with jelly and brown sugar and ketchup. Anjali's nose needed wiping; she looked dazed and kept her mouth open. Maya looked better, and hastily pulled her pajama top tightly around herself, suddenly conscious of the stranger's scrutiny. She patted down her hair and managed to streak it with flour. I was unshaven, and stood unsteadily in my magician's robe clutching a limp pancake.

"*Beautiful* family. Congratulations, you must be *proud* of them. *Beautiful!*"

We looked awful. We curled up and shrank.

"*Beautiful* family!" he repeated.

Mark Hastings beamed at Maya and the girls, and then turned to me.

"Doc, I need your help. My wife Amanda is real sick. She ate yesterday at Hidalgo's, you know, the Mexican place. She hasn't stopped throwing up since. I tried to give her some nausea pills I had from my knee surgery, but they didn't help. She just vomited then up as well. Thought of calling you at night, but figured you'd be sleeping so we toughed it out. But now, it's eight thirty, so I figured you'd be up and about, didn't figure you were fixin' to have breakfast."

"Your wife Amanda has been sick all night?" I asked.

"Yep."

"Where is she right now?"

"At home."

"Why didn't you go to the emergency room?"

He hesitated, looked away, and then looked back at me.

"Tell you the truth, Doc, Amanda doesn't like Karl Becker. And he's on call in the ER."

"Well, he's still on call. If you go to the ER, he will see you and take care of Amanda."

"That's the whole point, Doc, that's the whole point. *She doesn't want to see Karl!*"

"Why not?"

He shrugged.

"They just didn't hit it off. You know, different personalities. It happens. Anyhow, Doc, I'm asking you as a favor, a personal favor, to please see Amanda in the ER and take care of her."

I looked at Maya. She seemed confused. She shrugged her shoulders and threw up her hands and looked back at me. I didn't know what to say. Mark persisted.

"The docs here do it all the time. Doc Bulent, he comes to the ER and sees his own patients all the time, doesn't matter who's on call. Dr. Becker does it too, whenever he wants to."

"Yes, but Karl is on call. I think he should be the one to see her."

Mark sighed and sat down. He wiped his forehead and studied the carpet for a few seconds. I noticed his broad spade-like fingers and deeply tanned forearms. He clenched and unclenched his hands, then looked up.

"Doc, I don't want to get you crossways with Karl. You see, we're real good friends with the Templars. We were about to take Amanda to Abilene or Brownwood, but Tommy and Agatha Templar recommended you. We listen to them. They said you were good, and that's enough for us. If Amanda is staying in this town, then I want you looking after her, not Karl. If you won't help us, we're going to Brownwood or Abilene."

I sighed. Karl and Dr. Bulent certainly came in and saw their own patients whenever they wished, and I had no problem with that. It lessened my load, and I welcomed it. Karl occasionally saw his patients when I was on call, and Dr. Bulent invariably took over. I had been able to wriggle out of some early morning calls from the ER when they were Dr. Bulent's patients. *Check with Dr. Bulent and see if he wants me to see them, call me back if he wants me to see them.* I had never been called back in those cases.

"Mr. Hastings, let me—"

"Mark, call me Mark."

"Okay, yes, Mark. Let me do this. Let me call Dr. Becker and tell him that I would like to see your wife in the ER and look after her. I know that he has seen his own patients sometimes when I was the one on call. I don't really see why he should object, since it'll mean that he can stay in and rest at home and not have to come to the ER."

"You do that!" he nodded excitedly.

"I think that's fair."

I looked at Maya for confirmation but she was attending to the girls, hurriedly scrubbing their grubby faces with a wet towel.

"So *will* you see her in the ER?" he asked again.

"Yes, but I will also let Dr. Becker know that I am coming to see her."

"Good deal! See you in the ER in twenty minutes!"

"I'll see you there, Mr. Hastings. I mean, Mark."

"Doc, thanks a bunch. I appreciate this."

"You're welcome. See you soon."

"Adios!"

He tipped his hat at Maya, winked at the girls, and strode out. Outside, a truck sputtered and roared to life.

"Here, you can have this pancake. You had better get started! You're going to be late!" Maya said.

"Lucky we didn't have anything planned for this morning!" I said.

"We would have preferred you to be home with your family!" Maya looked at me and held my gaze. "You were a little quick to agree to see his wife and walk out on us."

I flushed. It was true.

"Yes, I was. I'm sorry. I guess I want to be just as successful as the other doctors, and the way to do that is to do favors."

There was an uncomfortable silence. I went on.

"Also, we need some letters of recommendation from the people of Hotspur for our green cards. I'm going to ask the Templars, of course, and if he's a friend of theirs, then he might write one as well."

Maya was mollified. She poured extra syrup on my pancake in forgiveness.

"I'm surprised he just came up to our front door and walked into our house."

"I was, too. But he seemed like a nice guy and he was sent by the Templars."

"And you need to build your practice. I know. So eat up and get going."

I dressed quickly and called Karl. His wife, Betty, answered.

"No, Sandy, Karl isn't at home. He may be running some errands or he may have gone to the hospital."

My heart sank. I didn't want Amanda and Mark to enter the ER, find Karl there, and tell him that I was taking charge. It was insulting for Karl to have someone familiar reject him in the ER and make other arrangements. It was more courteous if he heard it from me. I was sure I could present it in a way that he would understand. I tried him on his cell phone. No answer. I tried again. No answer.

"I'm sorry, but the person you're calling has a voice mailbox that has not been set up yet. Goodbye!" a voice announced cheerfully. The message started again the third time I tried and I hung up quickly.

I called the ER and asked for Karl. It was Gideon.

"Oh, he's not here, sir."

"Is he with a patient? On the floor?"

"Don't know. I can check. Hold, please."

After a few minutes Gideon returned.

"He was at the nurses' station, but he ain't there now. Don't know where he's gone."

I decided to talk to Karl as soon as I saw him.

"Well, if you see him, please tell him that I'm looking for him. I want to, ah, I *need* to talk to him. It's important."

"I got it, Doc!"

"Thanks! Also, I'll be coming in to see Mrs. Hastings. Would you call me when she gets there?"

"You mean Amanda Hastings? She's already here, Doc! You want to give me some orders?"

"She's already there? Has Dr. Becker already seen her?"

"Don't think so, Doc."

I was worried. I hurriedly said goodbye to Maya and the girls and drove down as quickly as I could. As I pulled into the parking lot, I noticed Karl's truck parked in a far corner. If I hadn't known it so well, I could have missed it. I wondered why he had parked so far away. Had he meant to go somewhere else? But it did mean that he was probably in the hospital somewhere. I hoped that he had not been in the ER when the Hastings arrived.

Amanda Hastings was sitting demurely sideways on the examination table. As I entered, she looked up and smiled. She offered me a manicured hand.

"Dr. Mathur? So pleased to meet you. *Amanda.*"

She looked stunning. She had blonde hair, tied up in a bun, a long neck, hazel eyes, and flawless makeup. A wave of verbena perfume scented her words and hung in the air. She wore a blue dress, pearl earrings, a pearl necklace, and a matching bracelet. I was taken aback.

"You don't look like my usual ER patient!" I blurted.

She smiled. I was surprised that she looked so good after throwing up all night.

"Doc, she got ready for this consult. Amanda's a real lady," Mark explained.

Amanda coughed impatiently. She dramatically raised the back of her hand to her forehead and exhaled loudly. The nurse stepped back, out of the limelight.

"I've been *so* sick!"

She shook her head and Mark leaned forward with a handkerchief.

"Thank you. I've been *so* sick!"

She looked at me imperiously. I didn't know my line and stammered, so she shrugged and went on.

"I ate at that awful place yesterday and I should have known better."

"Known better," Mark agreed.

"I had their fajitas," she explained. "Their shrimp fajitas."

Mark shook his head in disgust. Amanda pouted.

"Dr. Mathur, let me tell you something. Never trust seafood if you're in the heart of Texas!"

"I understand."

"Mark had the beef fajitas and he's fine. It was the shrimp fajitas. And of course we can't say a thing because Mark here, Mark here who's everyone's *favorite*, everyone's *buddy*, knows Hector who runs the place. So what are we going to do about it? Absolutely *nothing!*"

Mark half-grinned with his back to Amanda.

"Mrs. Hastings, Mark told me that you had a lot of nausea and vomiting. I take it you've been having that all night?'

"Yes, it was terrible. And oh, the diarrhea! The diarrhea has been terrible!"

"How many bowel movements have you had?"

"I can't say. I lost track. Maybe ten."

"Any fever?"

"No, I checked with a thermometer."

"Any blood in your stools?"

"No."

She turned her head and covered her face with her hands.

"Let me get a little history, Mrs. Hastings."

"Amanda."

"Yes, of course. Amanda, are you on any medication?"

"Occasionally I take Zyrtec for allergies. No prescriptions."

"Any allergies to medications?"

"Penicillin. It breaks me out. Makes me deathly sick. And what was that other one that *he* gave me?"

"Keflex."

"Yes, Keflex. Don't *ever* give me Keflex. Makes me feel like I can't breathe."

She exchanged knowing looks with Mark.

"You can tell him."

Mark shrugged.

"What happened was that Dr. Becker prescribed Keflex for Amanda and she was already known to be allergic to penicillin."

"*Highly* allergic!"

"Highly allergic to penicillin. She had a bad reaction to the Keflex and the pharmacist, Clem Haseltine, he goes to our church, you see, told us it should never have been given."

"Well, there is a thirty percent cross-reactivity," I explained. "Keflex is a different class of antibiotic, called a cephalosporin. But there is some cross-reactivity with penicillin."

"We know that, Doc. We looked it up. Still, I think he should have used something else."

I nodded silently. *This had probably been a simple oversight. The majority of patients with allergies to penicillin can tolerate cephalosporins but a sizable minority cannot.* I didn't want to prolong the discussion.

"What kind of operations have you had, Amanda?"

"I had my appendix out when I was six."

"I see. So that would be ten years ago?"

She laughed.

"You're just making *fun* of me."

But she kept smiling.

"Any other medical problems? Eye diseases, sinus problems, you mentioned allergies, any serious heart or lung diseases?"

"No, none."

"Ever been diagnosed with a stroke? Any severe migraines, headaches, fainting or loss of consciousness?"

"No."

"Diabetes, high cholesterol? Any problems with anxiety or depression?"

"I had slight diabetes during my first pregnancy."

"But not afterward?"

"No."

"Sometimes mothers become diabetic during pregnancy, but they usually go back to normal afterward. Usually if there is no major reason to have diabetes it does not come back."

"I was a little overweight at that time but I lost that weight and never put it back on." She jutted her chin up and looked away.

"Excellent. Now, I'm going to examine you."

I looked at her mouth with a pocket flashlight. Her mouth was dry and her saliva sticky, indicating dehydration. I noticed lipstick marks on her teeth.

"The lipstick marks on the outer surfaces of your teeth are still there and the lining of your mouth is very dry. You're definitely dehydrated."

I pinched her skin gently and let go. It flattened out slowly, another sign of dehydration. Her heart sounds were normal but her heart rate was rapid, around ninety per minute. Her lungs were clear. I had her lie flat and palpated her abdomen.

"Your liver and spleen are normal, but you feel very warm. Are you sure you don't have a fever?"

"Not when I checked it at home."

I completed my examination with a quick review of the nervous system. I checked for sensation and then the reflexes. She giggled as her knees jerked.

"Everyone tries to suppress them, but they still work. That's because they are reflexes and not really under the control of your brain."

The nurse checked her vital signs.

"Her blood pressure is ninety-four over seventy, pulse ninety-four, respirations eighteen and her temp is a hundred and one!"

"Is that bad?"

"You shouldn't have a fever. Uncomplicated gastroenteritis is usually afebrile, that is, there should *not* be a fever. You may have something more significant, like a bacterial infection."

"Like what?"

"Salmonella and Shigella are the common causes. Other bugs are Campylobacter and Yersinia. They can cause you to pass bloody stools as well."

Amanda was alarmed and reached out for Mark.

"What should we do?"

"Your vital signs are consistent with dehydration and possibly a bacterial gastroenteritis. I think we should admit you for rehydration and IV antibiotics. You should feel better soon enough."

"Can I go home tomorrow?"

"Maybe, maybe not. Depends on how you're doing. Why do you ask?"

"I teach in school and need to be back on Monday."

"Don't worry, Mandy, they'll get somebody," Mark murmured soothingly.

"Precious Mark! Precious, *precious* Mark!"

Mark took her hand and rubbed it.

"I'm going to write out the admission orders."

"Doc, do you think she should go to Abilene or Brownwood?" Mark asked.

"She should be just fine right here, Mark. It's pretty straightforward. But if you'd be more comfortable there, I'll be happy to transfer."

Mark turned to look at Amanda.

"What say, Precious?"

Amanda looked at me, paused, then spoke deliberately.

"Agatha Templar says you're good."

She swallowed hard and continued.

"If you're even half as good as she says, you should be good enough. I'll stay."

"Whoop!" exclaimed Mark, "You done good, Doc. If you can get *Amanda* to trust this hospital, you can get *anyone*."

I suddenly felt uncertain. Amanda had *high maintenance* written all over her. *Had I bitten off more than I could handle?*

"I really don't mind transferring you."

I was suddenly hoping she would agree.

"No transfer. I've made up my mind. I'm staying!"

We arranged a bed and transferred Amanda Hastings to the medical floor. The nurses came over and fussed.

"Amanda! Amanda Hastings! Lordy! Haven't seen you since Thanksgiving."

"How's Kevin?"

"Doing well. Works for the electric co-op now. How's your son?"

"Fine, just fine. He's at Tech. Wants to major in business."

"Fine school! Fine school!"

More nurses scuttled in and out.

"Wanda's going to be your nurse. I think you taught her daughter third grade English!" Gideon said.

"Honey, I *tried* to teach her."

Amanda was a local celebrity. The tumult made me forget about Karl. As the ER room emptied out, Gideon grabbed my sleeve. His eyes were wide and he spoke in a whisper.

"You finally got one with insurance, Doc!"

I said nothing.

"Doc, you know who that is?"

"Yes, it's Amanda Hastings. She's the science teacher in the school."

"No, I mean her husband. You know him?"

"No. Does he work in the school as well?"

"He's Mark Hastings, the biggest rancher around here. Owns thoroughbreds. Oil leases! Knows *everyone!* Knows the state representative. Knows the senator. Knows the *governor.*"

"I didn't know that."

"You did good today, Doc."

"How come?"

"If he likes you, he will tell everyone about you," Gideon explained. "Then maybe you get your green card and do well here. Real well!"

Gideon paused and then added, "Doc Becker called. Wants to talk with you. He's in his office. In the clinic."

"Does he know about Amanda? And my seeing her?"

"Yes."

My heart sank. The thrill of the morning collapsed and was replaced with a dark foreboding. I nodded and walked out. I headed up to the clinic, dreading my meeting with Karl. *I tried to inform him.*

The clinic was in semi-darkness. I swung the door open and called out. I walked into the waiting room and turned on the lights. The door to the nurses' station was open. Karl stood there, with something in his hands. He startled when he saw me. He dropped whatever he was carrying and charged into the waiting room to confront me. He was furious. His face shone with anger and his features were contorted. His eyes blazed and he spat out words like venom.

"What the *fuck* are you doing?"

"What do you mean?"

"What the *fuck* are you doing, you fucking shit?"

"Don't talk to me like that!"

"You stabbed me in the back! I've *always* supported you! And you? You had no business admitting Amanda Hastings! *I'm* on call! She shoulda come to *me!* You had no fucking business admitting her!"

"Her husband came to my home! He asked me to see Amanda as a personal favor!"

"So what about *me?* It makes me look like shit! They don't trust *me*, but they trust *you!* They don't get to choose! *I'm* on call, they all come to *me!*"

"Karl, when I'm on call, you and Dr. Bulent come and see and admit whomever you want to. I'm doing the same thing."

"You don't give a flying fuck what happens to this town! You're just here to get your damn visa! As soon as you get your damn green cards you and your family will get the hell outta here! And folks like me will stay here trying to help the locals!"

I was speechless. I was overcome with anger. I had done everything to make this work, I had always been polite to Karl, I had humored him and had never complained to him when he saw my patients. But I wanted to be a success too, I wanted patients to like me and come and see me, and I hated to always be submissive to Karl. I yelled back, and my voice boomed in the empty floor.

"Who the hell do you think you are? Who the hell are you to talk to me like that? Mark Hastings walked into my house this morning and asked me to see his wife, said they didn't want you. They were going to Abilene or Brownwood if I didn't see them!"

"So any dipshit comes to your house and tickles your tits and all of a sudden you're best buds? I shoulda been the one seeing his wife in the ER! I shoulda been the one to admit her. Not you!"

"She didn't *want* to see you. She was angry with you for giving her Keflex. She reacted to it and maybe that's why she's upset with you."

"I don't care," Karl yelled. "*I don't fucking care!* I always supported you and you stabbed me in the back. I get to see all the charity cases and the no-pays, but you just come in and take the cream of the crop. What gives you the right to see the big shots and leave all the others for me? Why don't you take *all* the calls?"

I gritted my teeth.

"Karl, I take the same calls as you. Calm down. You're making a big deal out of nothing."

"Am I? *Am I?* Ask yourself, how would you feel if you were in my shoes?"

"I tried to call you, to get your permission. Ask Betty."

"I don't give a rat's ass!"

"I tried calling you on your cell three times," I said. "Why didn't you answer?"

"I don't care! All I know is, you're a back-stabbing piece of shit!"

"I can't talk to you, Karl. Not like this."

"That's right! Just run away! Run off to your precious family! See if I protect you anymore! See if there's a burning cross on your front yard when you get home! Don't you fucking blame me!"

I stormed out, my face blazing with fury.

———————

On Sunday evening I was in Amanda's room, talking to her and Mark. She rested in bed, wore an elegant velvet robe over her hospital gown, and covered her feet with a leopard-print blanket. The room smelled of flowers and vanilla. There was a profusion of bouquets on the table and some even on the air conditioner. I examined her again; the signs of dehydration had resolved and she was afebrile. I checked the IV fluids and sat down on a stool next to her.

"The regional lab called me and said that Amanda's stool specimen will probably be positive for salmonella."

"Whoa! Salmonella! That's heavy-duty stuff!"

"But we got it in time. I started Amanda on IV Cipro and the bug is usually sensitive to that agent. Cipro has no similarity to penicillin, by the way. And there's no fever now. That's a good sign."

"So when can I go home?" Amanda asked.

"Let me get the reports tomorrow and check them. If there is good sensitivity to Cipro you could probably go home tomorrow on oral Cipro rather than IV."

"But will that be too soon? Will the oral Cipro be as good as the IV stuff?" Mark asked.

"Actually, yes, it should be. Cipro has excellent oral absorption and so we can safely change to the oral form without losing too much ground."

"Doc, we really appreciate what you've done for us," Mark said.

"Glad to be of help."

I examined the IV tubing and found an air bubble.

"Amanda, I'm going to flush the line. There's a small amount of air trapped here, so I'm just going to let it out."

I cleaned my hands and the tubing connection with alcohol, closed the valve above and disconnected the infusion. I opened the valve and let the saline and air bubble run out into gauze and then reconnected it. It ran smoothly.

"Dr. Mathur, I'm a science teacher," Amanda said. "I'm curious. What would happen if the air went inside me?"

"Well, a small amount of air would not do much. It would get mixed in with your blood, churned by the heart and absorbed or exhaled. But if there was a lot of air that got into your veins then that would be a serious problem. It could cause a blockage in your circulation."

"But air has a lot of oxygen and that gets absorbed, does it not?"

"Yes, but air is only twenty percent oxygen and almost eighty percent nitrogen, And nitrogen does not get absorbed, so it stays as a gas, like a bunch of balloons, in your bloodstream, and can get jammed. But that's rare."

"Have you ever seen it?" Amanda asked.

"Twice. Both were obstetric emergencies," I explained, "you know, during childbirth."

"And the drip you're giving me, what is that? I hope you don't mind all my questions."

"Not at all. The fluid you are getting is D5NS. The D stands for Dextrose, which is glucose, a sugar, and the 5 is for five percent, which means that there are five grams of it in one hundred milliliters of water."

"And the NS is for normal saline?"

"Correct. The NS stands for Normal Saline."

"That's my question. I figured that the NS was normal saline, but what do you mean by *normal*?"

Mark weighed in.

"I always figured it meant the ordinary kind of salt, you know, sodium chloride, as opposed to say, potassium chloride," he said.

"Actually normal saline means saline, sodium chloride, at the concentration that is safe to be mixed in with blood," I explained.

"I thought it was always safe to give saline."

"Saline *has* to be only *one* particular concentration. It has to be 0.9 percent, that's 0.9 grams in one hundred milliliters of water; otherwise the cells will either burst or shrivel. If the saline is too concentrated, the cells dry out and they shrivel. If the saline is too thin, the cells absorb water and they burst."

"Amazing! So saline could destroy all our blood cells?" Amanda asked.

"If it were the wrong concentration."

"So if you wanted to kill someone, you could give him or her the wrong kind of saline?" she asked.

"Yes, it's possible."

"Oh, I'm going to keep a close eye on Mark. He might see this as his big opportunity!"

"Yeah, Doc! That was a mistake, to tell me that! Mandy, you're a goner," Mark said with a broad grin.

They laughed.

"Saline! So much science in salt water!" Amanda remarked.

"I think it's fascinating that seawater has a similar concentration of salt—sodium chloride—and water," I said. "Makes me think there's a connection, you know, and it makes sense, because, after all, we all evolved that way. We evolved from fish, through amphibians, reptiles and then birds and mammals. So it makes sense that the salt and water in our blood reflects the sea, from where we all evolved."

Amanda and Mark looked at each other and were silent.

"Doc, I wouldn't say all that if I were you. See, lots of folks here don't believe all that evolution stuff. They believe in Intelligent Design," Amanda said, quietly.

I was taken aback.

"You don't believe in evolution?" I asked, astonished.

"Doesn't matter what I believe or don't believe, Doc. Folks here are good, respectful, God-fearing folks and *they* believe in Intelligent Design."

"So they believe that God created everything deliberately," I countered.

"Yes. God made us, Doc! God made us! That's what we believe!" Mark said, vehemently. He stood up and clenched and unclenched his fists.

I was quiet. Amanda spoke up.

"Doc, it's possible that you don't agree with Intelligent Design. But let's agree to disagree on that one, okay? Just let it be."

"I know we can't agree on every possible thing. I'm just learning to adjust and change. I guess we all need to adjust and change to circumstances. Sure, we can agree to disagree."

I turned to leave. I was irritated.

That's not true! I believe in evolution. I can't believe I'm too scared to speak up! Am I so desperate to get along? To build my practice at any cost?

Then a curious thought struck me.

I'm adapting to change. I'm learning to accept another point of view and that would give me a better chance of survival. I'm evolving by withholding my opinions—on evolution!

Mark coughed.

"Also, we heard about your, ah, *disagreement* with Dr. Becker," he said.

I was surprised and couldn't hide it. Mark smiled.

"Doc, this is a small town. Everyone knows everything. Always best to be honest here, cause folks usually know the answer when they ask you a question. Kind of like a good lawyer. We heard all about it through the grapevine."

"Yeah, Dr. Becker wasn't too happy," I said. "He has a different point of view, I guess."

"You know he wants to be Man of the Year?"

I paused.

"I'm on the committee that decides," Mark said.

"Maybe he wanted to look after Amanda to make you see him in a new light."

"Maybe. What do you think, Doc? You know you're the one who's going to nominate him."

"Well, I'll tell you. Karl has been good to me, and he has supported me. I'm going to continue to support his nomination. I think he's a good doctor."

Mark and Amanda looked at each other and nodded.

"What goes around comes around, Doc," Mark said. "Best to adjust. That's the ones that survive, the ones that adjust."

"You mean, survival of the fittest?"

Amanda jumped in, smiling.

"Oh no, Doctor, he didn't say that."

Karl called late Sunday night.

"Hey, Sandy, I'm really sorry I went off the deep end. I was frustrated with the Hastings, I guess. I've been doing everything to help them, but I just can't figure out Amanda."

"I understand. Karl, I really did try to reach you."

"Yeah, I've had phone problems. I guess if we had been able to talk then all this wouldn't have happened. You would have told them that Amanda had to see me, no choice."

I hesitated. I wasn't so sure I would have said that.

"Let's start afresh. Let bygones be bygones. Deal?"

"Deal!" I said, trying to sound sincere.

We discussed our families, the weather, and plans for the holidays. But the vision of an enraged Karl haunted me for days. And what had he been holding? It was a small, narrow cylinder, like a pen or a syringe. His face had been purple with anger, and his words had been full of malice. *A burning cross on my yard?*

I tried to ignore those memories at home but they flooded back in the clinic. I couldn't forget, even though I tried to offset it with all the times he had been helpful and kind and generous. We had declared a truce, but I knew it wasn't really over.

CHAPTER FOURTEEN

Seizure

Things changed after that. There was a lot of tension between Karl and me. For the first few weeks, Karl would jump to his feet and leave as soon as I entered the clinic. Later, he would stop in mid-sentence and glare silently at his coffee until I left, whereupon he would continue. He avoided talking to me completely for two weeks and, after that, only mumble or grunt monosyllables. The office staff sensed it immediately and grew wary. Laughter vanished and was replaced by a brittle politeness. Long silences replaced the chatter, and faces remained lowered and unwilling to engage.

At least, it was that way when I was around.

"Well, *obviously* they're going to support Karl. He's been there for years. He knows them all so well," Maya reasoned when we discussed the situation at home. "Just be patient. It'll pass."

But it didn't. It persisted for weeks. Karl would occasionally relent and smile: it was as if the sun had peered through the storm clouds and there was hope again. But, just as quickly, he would withdraw, and the spell would be broken, leaving only disappointment and a yearning for the way things used to be. I was at once impressed and resentful that Karl's whimsy controlled us so completely. I was reminded of other doctors I had antagonized. *I seem to irritate my colleagues. Maybe they find me stuck-up or lazy or something. I do get along with most of them, but the others really hate me!*

One thing did change. I started getting some patients from the public elementary school. Amanda Hastings and her husband recommended me to several of their colleagues, and a steady trickle of patients started coming in from the school. This had the effect of irritating Karl even more, and served as a constant reminder of my supposed infidelity. Sometimes they would wish him well if they walked past him in the office, and he ignored them. Some of them found the pressure to be too much.

"Doctor, I sure did appreciate you, but I've got to switch back to Dr. Becker. See, he goes to my church and now even teaches Sunday school. Can't help it, Doc," Homer Teegarten, the principal, told me.

There was nothing I could do about that. But others stuck with me and seemed to find Karl's attitude childish. Some of them would criticize him during office visits. I secretly wanted to encourage them, but realized it was mean-spirited. I remembered that, in a small town, everyone found out everything. I knew that Karl would eventually find out everything I said about him, so I always spoke positively about Karl's abilities. I hoped that it would get back to him and help heal the rift.

Six weeks later I was sitting in the office by Heather's desk, sipping my third cup of coffee, when Kendra wheeled around.

"Dr. Mathur, are you on call for the ER?"

"Yes."

"The ER has a patient. Clayton Barlow. He's in with—"

"Epilepsy," Heather said, without looking up.

Kendra nodded.

"He's always in with epilepsy. Only, no one can ever prove it or disprove it. He comes up and says he has had seizures, but no one has ever seen him have one. Dr. Becker thinks he's faking it," she elaborated.

"He wants to claim disability," added Heather, drily.

"Why don't we send him to a specialist?"

"Dr. Becker sent him to a neurologist in Abilene. He didn't show up. Said he had a seizure in the car on the way to see him. Second appointment, same thing. Third appointment, Dr. Becker told him that he was going to fire him if he didn't show up, so he showed up. Two hours late, and the specialist refused to see him."

I pounced.

"So he's *Karl's* patient? We should let him know. Maybe Karl would like to see him in the ER?"

Kendra and Heather exchanged glances and thought it over for a minute, then shook their heads simultaneously.

Heather announced, "Dr. Becker fired him. He doesn't want to see him anymore. He told us both a couple of times."

"Well, I just don't want to upset Karl. *Again.* Should we run it by him?"

Kendra shrugged and got up. She walked to the nurses' station and walked into an examination room. She returned within an instant.

"He says, go ahead and see him. Call him if you need help."

I could call Karl if I needed help. I took that as a good sign. Perhaps Karl was thawing.

━━━━━━

Clayton Barlow was sitting in a chair when I entered. He struggled to get up, gave up, and sat down again with a groan. He was a tall, thin man, bald, with a full beard, and wore large dark glasses. He had baggy jeans, suspenders, and an open shirt over a vest that said *Believe*.

He extended his hand weakly and said, "Excuse my laziness. Clay Barlow."

I smelt bacon. I noticed a white paper bag with grease stains.

"Good to meet you. I'm Dr. Mathur."

He regarded me for a moment.

"Dr. Mathur, I heard you're good. I need a good doctor. I'm sick! Real, real sick!"

I read his paperwork.

"You've got to help me," he said. "No one can figure out what's wrong with me!"

"Well, it says you're forty years old, single, smoke a pack of cigarettes a day, and have never had any surgery. You don't take any medicines and you're not allergic to anything. No family history of anything serious. Currently, you're unemployed."

"There is a family history, my grandpa had seizures. Can't get no job cause I got seizures. Real bad seizures."

"You had a seizure today?"

"Yep!" he said, triumphantly.

"Do you remember what happened?"

"Kind of. Guess I just went crazy and blacked out."

"Where did this happen?"

"The diner."

"What were you doing there?"

"Breakfast."

"You were having breakfast?"

"Yep. Eggs and bacon."

"Did you choke on your food?"

"Nope."

"Had you started eating or did it happen midway or after you finished?"

"Don't know, Doc. Maybe afterward."

"Did you feel weird before you had the attack?"

"I guess."

"Do you remember what you ate?"

"Nope."

"What's the last thing you remember?"

"Walking into the diner."

"And then what do you remember?"

"Eating, then I got crazy and had a seizure. Then woke up here."

"You don't remember anything in between?"

"Nope."

"What about the other attacks?"

"Don't remember nothing. Just a big blackout."

"What about your friends? Or family? Anyone witnessed an attack?"

"My family never has seen me have a seizure."

"When you recover, do you find that you've wet yourself or soiled yourself?"

"What?"

"Do you find you have passed urine or had a bowel movement? When you were unconscious?"

"Oh, that. Nope."

"Do you wake up to find that you're weak in an arm or leg?"

"Weak all over."

"Have you had any other problems with your nerves before?"

"I guess."

"Like what?"

"I feel tired all the time. Just so tired!"

"Any double vision? Any weakness of your face?"

"Nope."

"Any bad headaches?"

He suddenly perked up.

"Headaches? *Lord*, I got headaches! Terrible! Would *kill* a lesser man!"

I was getting nowhere with the seizures, and now this complication.

"Are your headaches in the front or back of the head or all over?"

"All over!"

I turned away, frustrated. His history was too vague. I could not tell from his account whether he had epilepsy. The evidence of a witness was essential. Grand mal seizures are very dramatic and an eyewitness account can clinch the diagnosis. Ben was the nurse in the ER that day.

"What's the problem, Doc?" Ben asked.

"I need a witness. If he had a grand mal seizure, then he would have fallen to the ground unconscious and had tremendous shaking of his arms and legs. No one would mistake that."

"Sounds violent!" Ben said.

"Yes. But if it were petit mal or minor epilepsy then the seizures can be very subtle. They can look like the person is just zoned out for a few minutes. It can be hard to tell."

"Well, we can call the restaurant," Ben said. "The waitress there should have seen the whole thing."

"That's what I thought! Call her for me."

We called the restaurant and tracked down the waitress. Everyone had heard of the event and the waitress had already regaled several patrons. She was pleased to relate it to me.

"Well, Clay had his eggs and bacon. Then he had his coffee. Then he asked for extra bacon."

"Then what happened?"

"He asked for more bacon to go."

"No, I mean, tell me about the seizure."

"He looks at me and closes his eyes and says, Louise, I'm gonna have a seizure. Then he grabbed his plate and threw it on the floor. Then he threw his coffee cup, then the water pitcher and the cutlery."

"He just started throwing things?"

"Yeah, went crazy, like I said."

"But were his arms and legs jerking? Did it look like he was having a seizure?" I asked.

"Just looked kinda crazy to me. But I didn't keep looking. I ducked. Boy, he made a *mess!*"

"Then he collapsed on the floor?"

"No, he just sat down again and put his head in his arms and went real quiet, kind of went to sleep."

"Did he jerk or move his arms or legs after the seizure, or whatever it was?"

"No. Just fell asleep."

"Was there any shaking of his hands or feet? Even a little?"

"Naw. Looked like he was resting."

"How was he before the attack?"

"Usual. Cutting up with the women, making jokes. Usual."

"When the paramedics arrived, did they have to clean out his airway? I mean, did they have to suck some food or liquid out of his throat?"

"He would have fought that," the waitress explained, "but he laid down on the stretcher nice and easy."

"By himself?"

"Surely."

"So he was sitting at a table, eating his breakfast when all this happened?"

"Well, actually he was at the counter."

"Did he fall down off the stool?"

"Nope."

"You might not have seen, but what about strange movements of his eyes?"

"Nope."

"Any change in his mood or his speech?"

"Nope. He spoke afterward, normal."

"What did he say?"

"Louise, I want my extra bacon. Took it, too."

I remembered the white paper bag with grease stains. *So he had this unusual seizure and remembered to take the extra bacon?*

"He didn't bite his tongue or pass urine or have a bowel movement?"

"Not with the attack. Thank God. We'd still be cleaning up."

I turned. Clay had the white bag in his hand and was finishing the bacon. He chewed the last rasher slowly and crushed the bag. He licked his lips and wiped them with the back of his hand. He cooly returned my incredulous expression and shrugged.

"Bacon is bacon."

He wiped his fingers on the bag, crushed it into a ball, and threw it into a corner.

"You heard of Bonnie and Clyde?"

I was completely confused.

"See, the famous gangster Clyde Barrow was my grandpa. He had seizures. We all got seizures. Runs in the family, seizures. You know something?"

He leaned forward and lowered his voice.

"Only reason they got him was on account of he had a seizure, drove his car into a tree. Then them Rangers pumped him and Bonnie full of lead! Rangers say they ambushed him and shot him and Bonnie, but that's not what really happened. People who was there, they know. Now the Rangers, they don't want you to know the truth, and the truth is, he was getting away and they'd have lost him, but he had this seizure and lost control. Call them Kill Barrow seizures!"

"But you're Barlow, not Barrow," I remarked.

"Had to change our name, we did, on account of them he killed. *Hundreds*, actually."

I paused to regroup. My mind was reeling. So maybe this was an *inherited* disorder? *Bonnie and Clyde?* This was becoming unbelievable. I racked my brain. *Huntington's disease?* No, it did not fit. I couldn't put it all together. There had been no symptoms or signs preceding the attack, and it certainly had been a very unusual attack. I was beginning to doubt that it had even been an attack. I couldn't find any features to suggest a genuine seizure. I resisted that conclusion because I wanted Karl to be wrong. I wanted to dramatically discover a case of atypical epilepsy that he had missed all along, and what if, what if, it really was the reason a famous gangster had been killed years ago? I was amused at my own pettiness: I was polite to Karl but really wanted to bring him down a notch.

Ben crept up and whispered.

"Mr. Abbott just called. He wants to see you when you have a minute."

I nodded. That was unusual. I wondered if it was about my salary again. I knew that most of the patients I had seen were in the ER rather than the clinic, had no insurance, and were not able to pay. John Abbott had hinted darkly that they made no effort to pay, either. *We need paying patients,* he was going to say, *or we can't pay you.* It could wait.

"I'm going to examine you," I said to Clay.

I went through the physical examination carefully. The general exam revealed a gaunt man with nicotine-stained fingers and beard, poor oral hygiene, eight remaining teeth, muffled heart sounds, and scattered wheezing in his lungs. His abdomen was soft and unremarkable. I focused on his neurological system. In London, I had taught myself how to do a quick but comprehensive neurological assessment. In the certification exam of the Royal College of Physicians, the British equivalent of Board Certification in the United States, we were required to perform such an evaluation in two minutes in front of two examiners. I had practiced it so many times that I could do it confidently. I stepped in front of Clay.

"Any change in your sense of smell?"

"Naw."

"Any blurred vision?"

"Nah."

"I'm going to look inside your eye. Just look straight in front."

I peered into his eye with an ophthalmoscope. It had taken me months to master the instrument, and I had realized that I must hover extremely close to my patient to be able to focus on the retina. Every time the red field came into view, I felt a thrill. *I was looking directly at a part of the brain!* The retina is a layer of nerve cells called rods and cones, and is sensitive to light. Wispy arteries and veins course over it, tapering as they get to the edges. I followed them carefully, looking for irregularities in their outlines and for small bleeds. I was so close to his face I could smell bacon and cigarettes.

Normal so far.

"Follow my finger with your eyes, your eyes only, don't move your head."

The eyes moved in all directions and remained coordinated. The pupils responded appropriately to light and adjusted for distant and close objects.

"Can you feel this on your face?"

I touched his face in different places with a cotton swab. No loss of sensation. I shone a flashlight in his mouth and watched as he whisked his tongue dutifully and swallowed on command. I went over his reflexes rapidly and noticed that he winced. When I checked his strength, he was curiously passive.

"What's the matter? Can't you push any harder?"

"Guess I'm weak, Doc. *Pitiful* weak."

"Let me check for sensation. Do you feel me touching your hands?"

"Don't feel anything."

"How about here, on your chest? Can you feel this?"

"Nope."

"How about your legs? Can you feel me touching your legs?"

"You're touching my legs?"

"So you can't feel anything below your neck?"

"I guess."

I stepped back and wondered. I tried to suppress the feelings of disbelief that were gathering in my mind. I wanted to remain objective and gave him the benefit of a complete exam. I wanted to believe him, but with his supposed sensory loss, he would have to have severe damage to his spinal cord in the neck or a massive injury on both sides of the brain. *It did not make sense.* There was no history of trauma and he had a normal CT scan of his head two weeks ago in Brownwood.

"I'm going to run some blood tests," I announced. "While they're running, I'm going to see Mr. Abbott."

Clay slumped back in relief.

As I walked into the administration office, I was surprised to see Karl talking to Francisca. She was sitting bolt upright, and did not look at me as I entered.

Karl swung back and greeted me curtly, "Hey, Sandy."

"Hi, Karl. How are things?"

He shrugged.

"They just made me Man of the Year. Guess they ran out of folks to give it to."

"Congratulations!"

I smiled tightly. I was instantly envious, and I briefly regretted writing the nomination. With a struggle, I reminded myself of all the times Karl had helped me, and I suppressed my dismay.

"Yeah, whatever. John's going to ask you to make a little speech afterward."

"Of course!"

"How's our friend in the ER?" Karl asked.

"To tell you the truth, I'm confused. He says he had a seizure."

"I don't give a rat's ass what he says," Karl said, shaking his head.

"Well, I have my doubts."

"Did he tell you some tall tale?"

"He said he was related to Clyde Barrow."

"He's just full of it!"

"You don't think it might just be true?"

"Sandy, for a specialist in crap, you sure don't recognize it when you see it!"

My face burned. *Of course, Karl's right. That stuff about the gangster is ridiculous.*

"I may have to refer him to a specialist."

"Been there, done that. No good."

"What do you recommend?"

"What do I *recommend*? I recommend that you kick his sorry ass out!"

"But what if we're missing something? What if he does actually have epilepsy or something?"

"Are you *kidding* me? You really *believe* this guy?" Karl took a step back and stared at me with astonishment. I shrugged and sighed.

"Well, I find it difficult to believe him, but I want to find out what's really happening."

I *wanted* him to have epilepsy. Karl stepped forward and glared.

"You think you're this great specialist from London and Houston who's going to show these dumb country docs what idiots they are? How they missed the diagnosis of some rare kind of epilepsy?"

I opened my mouth to answer, but didn't.

"Don't bother to answer. Listen, majesty. Do you know the tuning fork test?"

"The tuning fork test?"

"Yeah. In your training in the Royal College in England, when you were an intern, or a pageboy, or royal rectal examiner or whatever, in all that training, did they not teach you the tuning fork test?"

"No."

He turned triumphantly to Francisca, shaking his head in mock disbelief.

"I don't believe it. He trained in London and Houston and was certified by the fancy-ass frilly shirted wig whammed Royal College of Physicians."

He faced me and took a deep breath. He studied my face for a few minutes, and exhaled.

"The tuning fork test, Dr. Watson. When you want to provoke an attack of epilepsy. When you want to bring out an attack of full-blown epilepsy, Watson, you advise the patient that, if there *really* is epilepsy, the tuning fork will bring it out. You bang a tuning fork till it buzzes like a cicada and then you place it on the forehead."

I stared at him in astonishment.

"And if there really is epilepsy, Dr. Watson, then the patient will have an attack of epilepsy right then."

I stared at him fixedly.

"There's no such test," I said.

Karl smiled slowly, nodding.

"You know my methods, Watson! Apply them!"

"So you're misleading a hypochondriac or malingerer?"

"Elementary, my dear Watson."

"But is it ethical?"

He shrugged and walked away.

"DKDC," Karl said, and walked to the stairs.

Francisca smiled helpfully.

"Don't know, don't care," she explained and tittered.

I watched Karl's retreating figure with confusion. *Is it ethical to try out the tuning fork test to unmask spurious epilepsy? Is it against the Hippocratic oath? Will I be harming the patient?*

"Oh, Dr. Mathur, there was a man here to see you. Mr. Abbott told him you were busy, so he left. I saw him go upstairs to the clinic."

"A patient?"

"Don't know. He gave Mr. Abbott his card, said his name's Torres. He went upstairs. That's why we were calling you."

Back in the ER, I confronted Clay. He sat on the side of the table, wiped his glasses and held them up to the light. He put them back on hurriedly and turned to me, and started to moan. I decided to go ahead. I rummaged in the cabinet and found a tuning fork. I decided to go in for a bit of showmanship. I turned around and held it up triumphantly, like an Oscar. Ben was surprised.

"Mr. Barrow—"

"Barlow!"

"Okay, Mr. Barlow. Have you seen a neurologist? You know, a nerve specialist?"

"Yeah."

"What have they told you?"

"They don't know *what's* happening!"

"Did they say you have epilepsy?"

"All they say is, we don't understand what's going on in that head of yours, Mr. Barlow, we don't know squat! Don't come back, because we can't help you, they say!"

"Maybe they *don't* think you have epilepsy?" I said.

"Nope. I got seizures, like my grandpa, and no one can tell me *nothing!*"

I took a deep breath.

"Then let me try to help. I am going to perform a very dangerous test. It is a test that may bring out epilepsy. In some people with a rare form of epilepsy, we can provoke an attack of epilepsy."

"What do you mean?" Clay said, suspiciously.

"I mean, if there *really* is epilepsy, we can make an attack of epilepsy happen."

"How?"

"With a tuning fork, like this one. I want to do this test for you to see if you really have epilepsy."

Clay looked startled. He glanced quickly at Ben, who, to his credit, remained impassive. Clay hesitated, then squared his shoulders.

"Just don't hurt me!"

"I won't."

"What do I do?"

"Just lie down on the table. Let me make sure your IV is working."

I checked his IV line. Ben had hooked him up to normal saline and it was dripping in slowly. I turned to Ben.

"Keep some diazepam ready."

"Yes sir. Got it right here, Doc!"

I addressed Clay gravely. He was starting to turn pale.

"Clay, I'm going to hit a tuning fork on a rubber pad. It will start to vibrate."

I picked up a tuning fork and smacked it hard. It buzzed like a chainsaw. Holding the fork by the stem, I walked briskly to Clay.

"Now I'm going to place it on your head, to see if it brings out the epilepsy!"

I placed the base of the tuning fork on the middle of his forehead. Then an incredible thing happened. He started to shake violently. He thrashed his arms and legs as if electrocuted, and his trunk heaved up and down, slamming the gurney. Taken aback, I stepped back, taking the tuning fork with me. The movements stopped instantly. Clay gave me a weak grin.

"Guess it worked, Doc!"

I stared at him incredulously. Emboldened, I struck the fork again and connected for a split second. Clay burst into spasmodic jerking again, but just as briefly. I did it again: the same result. Then I became reckless. I whacked the fork against the pad theatrically and placed the throbbing instrument on his right shoulder. The right upper limb alone convulsed. The same thing happened on the left shoulder. I stood back, shaking my head in disbelief.

Ben muffled his laughter.

"Do his elbow!" he urged.

I obliged.

The forearm and the hand writhed, as the rest of Clay's body remained immobile. Clay gazed in awe at his dancing forearm, then turned to me, dazzled by my display of medical brilliance.

"I reckon you figured it out, Doc! Man, you're the *best!*"

I placed the tuning fork on the base of a finger. The finger leapt into activity, curling and uncurling with vehemence. There was a guffaw behind me and Karl came bursting out.

"You damn fraud!"

Clay scanned our faces and rose angrily.

"You great big fraud!" Karl repeated, laughing.

"I got epilepsy!"

"No, you don't! There's no such thing as epilepsy due to a tuning fork, you fraud! You fell for it!"

Clay looked at me, and he slowly realized what had happened. His face screwed up in anger and he sat up abruptly. I smiled, triumphant but embarrassed. Clay leaped off the gurney and lunged for his belongings.

"Screw you all! Screw you!"

He retreated to the corner.

"Fraud!" Karl boomed.

"Where you going?" Ben demanded. "You got some answering to do, partner!"

Clay gave a tug on his IV and yanked it out. Watery blood splattered the floor. Ben spun around to grab paper towels. Clay saw his chance and bolted, pushing past both of us. Karl hurled the discarded bacon bag at him.

"Bacon is bacon, and fakin' is fakin'!" he yelled after Clay.

"Restaurant wants forty bucks!" Ben hollered.

Karl and I went up to the clinic, still chuckling. Karl was pleased that I had taken his advice and put his arm on my shoulder. We laughed together, and it felt good to have our old camaraderie back. Heather was standing in the waiting room.

"Dr. Mathur, there's someone to see you."

"A patient?"

"Well, I don't know what it's about. He wouldn't say."

She glanced at Karl as if searching for a clue.

"He's in room three, Dr. Mathur."

Karl went for coffee. I strode into the examination room with a clipboard, beaming. I offered my hand.

"I'm Dr. Mathur. Sorry if I kept you waiting. Please, please sit down."

The man looked like a tubby schoolboy. He had a round face, happy brown eyes, and a mop of black hair molded by his Stetson, which he held to his chest with his left hand. He wore starched khaki trousers and a white shirt. A large silver belt buckle was inscribed, simply, LAW. He shook my hand vigorously but kept standing.

"Dr. Mathur, my name is Officer Enrico Torres. I work for the Texas State Board of Medical Licensure and the DEA. I'm conducting an inquiry into the death of one of your patients, Mr. Truman Sparky Cummins. You are hereby notified that you are under investigation."

CHAPTER FIFTEEN

Going for the Jugular

"What do you mean? Why are they investigating you?" Maya asked during dinner.

We were seated at the dining table. Maya had made spicy beans and potatoes, lentil soup, and basmati rice, but I had lost my appetite. Priya and Anjali were on their second helping while I toyed with my food. They looked up at us with concern and stopped eating. Anjali spilt some rice on the floor, and I snapped at her. Priya jumped off, swept it up with her napkin, and sat back silently. Maya stirred the rice, added some butter, covered it again, and fixed me with her gaze. I flinched and reached for the beans and potatoes.

"You look very worried. Is there something wrong?" Maya asked.

I added more food to my plate and started eating to avoid answering. Maya waited patiently and repeated the question. I sighed, put my spoon down, and drank some water.

"Why don't you answer?" my wife pressed. "Silence makes you look guilty!"

"What was your question?" I asked, testily.

"Did you do something wrong?" Maya asked again.

I had asked myself that over and over. I had replayed the investigator's sentences in my mind and had wondered whether I had indeed done something wrong. Part of my mind leapt to my defense, but there was concern. *Had I missed filling out the consent form? Had I dissuaded him from going to Abilene and seeking help elsewhere? Had I glibly talked him into staying in Hotspur so that I could have a patient? Was I intent only on proving I was competent?*

"I don't think so," I answered.

I looked at Maya. She was upset and worried, too. She looked at her plate, then fussed over the girls for a few minutes. She pursed her lips and rubbed her eyes.

"This affects everything, doesn't it?" she said, slowly.

"Yes," I answered.

"If they take away your license then there's no practice, no job, and no green cards, right?"

"Right. This is very big. We are halfway through the immigration process, the lawyer said, and we're at a critical stage. During the investigation, the application is held up and if it's held up too long, it'll be dropped."

I remembered being concerned about my Royal College tie and retrieving it from the trashcan. *Had I forgotten to write some details because I was distracted?*

"He said they could not find documentation that the patient had consented to stay in Hotspur, that he had been informed that he could have gone to Abilene or San Angelo or some other bigger city," I explained.

Anjali choked and spat up into her plate. I snapped at her again and she started crying. Priya wrapped an arm around her. Anjali bit her lip, then resumed eating without looking up. I regretted losing my temper and mumbled an apology. Priya kept her arm in place protectively.

"Why couldn't they find it?" Maya asked.

"I don't know."

"Is there a form?"

"Yes."

"Did you fill it out? Did he sign it?"

"I think so, yes."

"You *think* so? Something this important, you need to be *sure!*"

"Well, I'm pretty sure that I did fill it out. Only we can't find it in the chart."

"Was it misfiled? Could it be in another chart?"

"I don't know, damn it! I don't know where the hell it is!" I burst out.

Maya stiffened. Anjali started crying again and Priya wiped her eyes. She pushed back from the table.

"Eat your food!" I ordered. Maya leaned forward and stroked Anjali's face and spoke softly to the girls.

"It's okay. Daddy's upset because of something at work. Don't worry."

But they lowered their heads and refused to eat. We pleaded with them, and they picked at their food sullenly and kept their heads bowed.

"I don't know where the form is."

"So why don't they look in another chart?"

"They have already looked in all the charts of the patients admitted that week and the month before and after his death. It's not there."

Maya moved a platter of fruit and started peeling an apple. She stopped and stared at it thoughtfully.

"Could someone have *removed* it from the chart?"

"Possibly. I thought about it. But that's hard to prove."

"What about the patient's husband or wife or family?" she asked. She gave the girls slices of apple and they gnawed on them unhappily.

"The patient's wife was in the room all the time and we're trying to reach her. She would be the perfect witness. She would back me up, I'm sure of it. But for some stupid reason, she can't be reached."

"What do you mean?"

"Well, no one knows where she is. She doesn't have any family in town, and no one knows where her children live. She had her children before she met Sparky. Then they had a son together, but he died. Her name was Esperanza, and I think she's Hispanic. Don't know much more about her. He was the patient, not her."

"Does she have a hospital chart? There would be an emergency contact."

"I thought of that. All she had was an ER visit, and the only number listed was her husband's cell phone. And Sparky's dead. That number's no longer in service."

Maya handed out more apple slices. Priya and Anjali ate slowly and silently.

"Really, how big a deal *is* this?" Maya asked.

"This is a *very* big deal. The patient *died*. He was under my care, so I'm totally responsible for what happened to him before his . . . death. And they want to make sure that he knew what he was doing. They want some proof that he had been informed about his options."

"Didn't you write something in the notes?"

"Yes, I did. But they want to see something signed by him, or to speak to his wife."

"So you really need to find his wife."

"That's what I've been trying to do. I even called the police, and they went over to his—*her* house. It's all locked up, meters turned off, yard's all overgrown, house falling down. Sparky and Esperanza never talked to their neighbors. No one's home now."

"She can't just vanish."

"Well, she isn't at home and her cell phone is disconnected and no one knows where she lives or where her family or children are, so it's difficult."

"So what are you going to do?"

"I'm going to call the minister of her church and see if he has any information. Then I'll call the chief of police."

"Well, at least you have a plan."

We cleaned up quietly, and the girls helped load the dishwasher. Maya put the food away and looked thoughtful. Afterwards, I hugged Anjali and Priya and teased them about their inability to line up the cups and plates to fit everything into the dishwasher. They brightened up.

"How about a good-night story?" asked Priya.

I started to say no, then stopped. *It might be just the thing to get my mind off the day's events.* I had not spoken to them much, and I grasped the opportunity.

"Sure. How about an Akbar and Birbal story?"

"Yes!" they cried out and ran to change into their nightgowns and brush their teeth.

The girls tumbled into their beds. I turned the lights off and sat in the darkness with my back to the window. I sucked in the smell of freshly laundered linen and shampoo. The anger and resentment ebbed, and my mind calmed down. As I selected a story I wondered what my grandmother had thought as she selected stories. Did she think of *her* mother and grandmother? The girls tossed impatiently. I watched the shadows flung across the room as headlights swept past and waited for the rustling to stop and the girls to calm down. Eventually, their movement and chatter softened, then ceased, and I listened to them breathe. The moonlight silvered their faces and forms, like pharaohs. They turned expectantly.

"Hurry, Daddy!" Anjali said.

"I was waiting for you two to calm down," I said. "Are you ready for the story?"

"Yes!" they said in unison.

"Okay then. So you remember that the greatest Moghul ruler of India was . . ."

"Akbar!"

"Right! And his prime minister was a clever man called—"

"Birbal!"

"Right again. And Birbal helped Akbar figure out many difficult problems. Have I told you the one about the beggar and the woman selling fish? Well, okay. Once, there was a woman who used to fry fish and sell it in the market. One day, a beggar began sitting next to her."

"What's beggar?" asked Anjali .

"A poor man who has nothing and has to ask everyone to give him money," Priya explained. "Go on, Dad."

"Yes, a beggar is a poor man who has no money and he begs for money and other things from other people so that he can eat and live. The beggar sat next to the woman who was frying fish and ate whatever little food he had. Well, the woman who was frying fish got angry with the poor beggar."

"Why?" Anjali asked.

"She was angry because the beggar was smelling her fish. He was smelling her fish and enjoying the smell and it made him enjoy his food more. So the woman said, you owe me a copper coin, because you're enjoying my fish!"

"But he was only *smelling* it!" Priya protested.

"Right!"

I allowed the indignation to swell.

"That not fair!" they cried.

"So she went to a judge and no one knew what to do. So, eventually, the matter reached the royal court. Akbar asked Birbal to decide."

"What did Birbal say?"

"Birbal said that what the woman said was *true*, that the beggar *had* enjoyed his bread much more because he had smelt the fish frying. And he had *not* paid for the fish."

The girls groaned.

"So he asked them to all step back outside into the street. He gave the beggar a copper coin and told the woman to put her hand out for the coin. She did that, she put her hand out for the coin."

"*What?* Birbal just *gave* her the coin?" Priya asked.

I smiled.

"No, he didn't. He gave the coin to the beggar and told him to hold it up above the woman's palm so that its shadow fell on her palm."

I delivered the denouement.

"And he said that the right payment for *smelling* fish frying is the *shadow* of a copper coin!"

The girls loved it.

I smiled. Now *that's* justice.

─────────────

I wasn't able to sleep well. I kept going over the events of the day. I saw the investigator, standing up and shaking hands, grasping my hand firmly. *The snake!* I remembered his pleasant tone. *You're under investigation.* I had felt a flush of shame and guilt and tried hard not to blink and appear suspicious. I had offered, perhaps too zealously, to do everything I could to help with the investigation. I tried to explain my background in internal medicine and my years in London, but he had dismissed that. He was only interested in the facts and then he had to wrap up the investigation and "giddyup back to Austin pronto." They were short-staffed, he explained, and he was needed for many other cases as well.

My mind churned relentlessly, but I could not distill any new thoughts. *This can't be happening!* I kept trying to think clearly, but kept getting more upset. *This is insane*, I thought, *I have to go to sleep.* I wondered about taking Benadryl to help me sleep, then decided against it. Antihistamines always made me sleepy the next day as well, and I needed to be alert. The harder I tried to sleep, the louder the crickets chirped and the fan hummed. I listened to the hiss of the air conditioner, heard it pause, then start up again sluggishly. I heard the headboard tap the wall. I heard Maya breathe. *Everything irritated me.* I felt the sheets were too warm and angrily kicked them off.

It was almost a relief when the phone rang. I jumped and snatched it up.

"Dr. Mathur? This's Ben in ER. Are you still on call?"

"Yes."

"Sorry to bother. Got a frequent flyer. Tricia White."

He paused.

"You know Tricia White, don't you?"

"Not really."

"Well, drug and alcohol abuser, prostitute—I mean, *lady of the night*, you know what I mean."

"What's the problem?"

"She says she just doesn't feel well. Vitals okay, except she's running a fever of a hundred and one."

"That's significant. Is she doing IV drugs?"

"Doc, is the day long? Is the sun bright?"

"Okay, I get it. Let's get a CBC and a CMP and a sed rate."

These tests cover a wide set of diagnoses, including anemia, infection, and inflammation.

"Want a UA and chest X-ray?"

"Yes, good idea. Let's check her urine, could have a urinary infection causing her fever. I'll be there soon."

"Well, maybe you don't have to come. Maybe I can manage her and maybe discharge her and you can see her in your clinic in the morning?"

I hesitated. He was offering me a chance to stay home and sleep. Something about the story bothered me. I knew that intravenous drug abusers are at risk for several diseases, and they often lied about symptoms and manipulated their stories. I had seen many in London and Houston. Many sought narcotics, some even stole drugs from hospitals and ER rooms. Some kept injecting themselves with dirty needles and ended up with serious infections. And some had sued their doctors. *She's probably very sick, very poor and will have no hesitation in suing me.* I sat up on the side of the bed, looked at the floor, and sighed. The bitterness subsided.

"I'm coming. Ten minutes."

At two o'clock in the morning in rural Texas, the stars are breathtaking. As I stepped out to walk to my car the spectacle astonished me again. I stood in awe and took in the night sky, a gigantic black treasure box flung open, jewels scattered and glittering. *City dwellers had no idea of the magnificence of the night. Planet Earth, plunging through an expanding universe, hurtling on with millions of other stars, all exploding and collapsing, with dark matter and black holes! There's a galactic kaleidoscope churning above me, and here I am in a Toyota Corolla trying to remember the speed limit.*

Ben greeted me at the door to the ER. There was only his truck parked outside. Ben threw up his hands.

"Well, look-ee here! It's the doctor!"

"Hey, Ben! We have her labs back?"

"Not yet. Had to get Joe out of bed. He just got here, just getting ready."

Tricia White was sitting on the side of the examination table. She was a thin woman in her thirties, but looked older. Her face was streaked with mascara and thickly applied makeup and she wore bright green contact lenses. Tattoos of stars and armadillos covered her forearms and ankles. Her nose and lower lip were pierced and gave her a permanent pout. Her hair was black with green highlights, and her dress had a neckline that plunged in search of a cleavage. She lit a cigarette.

"No! Put that out!" Ben yelled.

Ben leapt and snatched the cigarette out of her hand.

"Screw you," she said calmly and turned to me.

She offered me her hand and announced, "Tricia White. Pleased to meet you."

I shook hands and sat down. I was amused and impressed by her calm demeanor. I reached for the clipboard and read aloud.

"You're Patricia White, thirty-six years old, single, and you live here in Hotspur."

"Guilty!"

Her voice was hoarse. She coughed into a paper napkin.

"You don't take any medicines? You have no allergies to medicines that you know of?"

"That I know of, correct. May I smoke?"

"I'm sorry, you can't smoke in the hospital."

"You call this a hospital?"

"Saved you many a time!" snapped Ben.

"Be quiet, sir. I'm talking to the doctor."

Ben scowled and turned away.

"Can't smoke cigarettes, can't smoke weed?" she asked.

I shook my head.

"You've never had any kind of surgery in the past?" I continued.

"Tonsils taken out when I was two. That count?"

"Yes. Anything else?"

"Nope."

"So what's the problem right now?"

She sagged forward and lowered her voice as if telling me a secret.

"I just don't feel well. I feel as if something's wrong, don't know what. Just feel *bad*."

She coughed again and brought up some clear sputum.

"I got a fever and I feel sick," she said. "I feel I could puke right now."

I took a step back.

"Any headaches? Neck pain? Muscle pains?"

"Just the usual."

"But anything new? Any chest pain, abdominal pain, or new pain anywhere in your body?"

"Nope. Just feel like crap!"

"Any blood in your urine? Dark colored urine?"

"Nope."

"Any changes in your bowels? Any diarrhea or constipation issues?"

"Same old, same old."

"Any illness run in your family?"

"I'm adopted."

"You still doing drugs?"

"Uh-huh."

"IV drugs?"

"Eh?" she looked at me, puzzled.

"I mean, are you injecting yourself? Through the veins?"

"Yeah. Sometimes."

"When was the last time?"

"Couple weeks ago."

"What about alcohol?"

"What about it?"

"Do you drink alcohol on a regular basis?"

She looked at me in surprise and threw her head back and laughed hoarsely, sounding like a fork scratching metal.

"I drink pretty regular! Six-pack a day!"

"Six-pack's the minimum," muttered Ben.

Ignoring him, Tricia leaned forward, squeezed my hand, and pleaded.

"Doc, I ain't kidding. I'm *sick*. There's something wrong, I ain't ever felt this bad. I know my body, there's something wrong. You think I'd be in this two-bit hospital at two in the morning when I could be working? Check with Mr. Ben there, I never come at night. I'm sick real *bad!*"

Ben turned away and busied himself with paperwork.

I reviewed her vital signs. She had a fever of a hundred and one degrees, but her blood pressure and pulse were normal. I examined her. She smelled of cigarettes and air freshener. Her skin was tanned and felt like canvas. There were little bumps over her veins, hillocks of fibrous tissue, scars from previous needling, nestled in her elbow and on her hands. I had seen this many times in addicts; more marks on the left, more damage on the right, because most are right-handed. She was pale. Her heart rate was rapid, and I thought I heard a soft murmur. Her lungs wheezed as expected. Her abdomen was normal. I examined her reflexes and checked for sensation. Her muscle strength was adequate, but she complained about muscle aching. I stepped back to the end of the bed and surveyed Tricia.

She drooped and did not look well.

A colleague in London had called it the end-of-the-bed-a-gram, and I surveyed her with concern. Her end-of-the-bed-a-gram was bad. Something was wrong, and I didn't know what. She wasn't like Clay Barlow, who had been faking seizures. She looked ill.

I realized that I ached all over. I was tired and angry and upset. I remembered why: the investigator, the investigation, the humiliation, the potential loss of the green cards. I cleared my mind with an effort.

"What about the labs?" I asked Ben.

"Joe's here. He's in the office behind you making the labels."

Joe slouched in without acknowledgment. He looked tired and avoided looking at Patricia and got straight down to business. He scanned both forearms and shook his head. He tied tourniquets and looked again, gently probing with his fingertips, hunting for veins. He moved the tourniquets and tried again. No luck. He spoke quietly to me.

"Try the feet?" Joe asked.

"Go ahead," I said.

He tied the tourniquet on one ankle, then the other. Once, he was enthused, but then shook his head. Too small, too crooked. He tried both sides, but there was nothing.

"Sorry. No veins anywhere, Doc!"

He stood up, unsure.

"We have to have blood tests," I said. "They're critical. I also need blood cultures times three. I'm worried she has bacterial endocarditis."

"What's that?" Joe asked.

"That's where bacteria get into the bloodstream because of IV drug use. They go and stick to the valves of the heart and grow there. They eat into the valves and keep dripping into the blood and spread all over the body."

"*Shit!* I have that?" Patricia looked alarmed.

"Maybe. That's my concern."

"Can you fix it?" she asked.

"Yes, with strong antibiotics."

"Do it! Do it! What're we waiting for?"

"We have to have an IV line, and Joe can't find a vein, probably because previous IV drug use has scarred them up. Joe's the best, and if he can't find a vein, then there isn't one to be found."

Joe grunted slightly at the compliment.

"So I think I need to start a central line," I continued.

"What's that?"

"I need to place an IV in a big deep vein so we can take blood samples and give you antibiotics."

"Where you going to put it?"

"I prefer to put it in your neck. It's the safest choice. I can also try the groin or under the collarbone, but the groin isn't clean and the vein under the collarbone is riskier."

"What're the risks?" she asked.

"Well, there are some significant risks. The biggest risks of this procedure are that you could bleed heavily and you could lose a lot of blood and have a big swelling in your neck."

"You mean, hematoma or blood clot?" Tricia asked.

"Yes."

"Heck, I've done that to myself, injecting myself! Bleeding? Survived it."

I grimaced.

"There is also the risk that I could hit the carotid artery that lies next to the vein. That's the artery that takes blood to your brain. If I hit it, you could have less blood going to your brain. You could have a stroke."

"Shit! Don't do that! I mean, go ahead and do the IV, just don't screw up my brain. Lord knows it's pretty screwed up already."

I handed her a form.

"Please read and sign this consent form."

Tricia reached for her purse and pulled out her glasses and put them on and read the form. I noticed she had many bottles of pills in her bag, besides cigarettes and keys and a lot of folded paper. She noticed.

"The papers? Articles I cut out. I like to read, believe it or not. When I find me a good article I read it over and over. Best way to remember something good. Repetition, repetition."

"I agree. Have you read the consent?"

She signed it and handed it back.

"Yeah. Here."

Ben helped me prepare her. Joe hunched down on a low stool like a buzzard and watched us.

"Doc Becker, *he* always places central lines in the groin," Joe muttered.

"I understand. I can do that, but looking after groin lines is a pain. They tend to get infected. A line in the neck is easier to look after."

"Doc Becker is a *really good* Doc and *he* puts them in the groin," Joe continued.

"Well, *I'm* more comfortable with the neck, so that's what *I'm* going to do."

"No risk of hitting the brain artery in the groin."

I looked up, irritated, then bit my lip and concentrated. I had Patricia lie flat and I sat on a stool near her head, so I could look straight down at her face and neck. I had her raise her chin and move it to her left, stretching her neck. I palpated the carotid artery just inside the big muscle of the neck, the sternocleidomastoid. I put on sterile gloves and cleaned her neck with alcohol, then with iodine. The pungent smell of iodine always reminded me of my nights on call in London, of placing these IV lines in emergency rooms, in ICUs, and even in X-ray departments. *I'm pretty good at them.* I reassured myself, *I've done this many times. I can do this.*

"Heard the State Board's here. Investigating you?" asked Joe pleasantly.

I looked up angrily. I was about to snap back, but stopped.

"Yes."

I draped her neck with sterile green towels and Ben focused the overhead light. I changed gloves and put on a gown and mask.

"Doc Becker don't need gown and mask," Joe noted.

I felt the carotid artery again with the fingers of my left hand. I picked up the syringe with lidocaine and looked up at Ben for confirmation.

"Five percent lidocaine with epi, just like you like it," he said.

I kept my left fingers on the artery and injected lidocaine with my right hand gently on the outer side of the artery, raising a bleb. Tricia lay still.

"You okay?" I asked.

"Fine."

"I've injected lidocaine. This is the numbing medicine. Now I'm going to place the IV. This may hurt a little. You're going to feel some poking around."

She grunted. She glanced at me; there was a flicker of concern, then she looked away. With my left fingers still on the artery, I picked up the intravenous catheter with my right hand and inspected it. It was a four-inch hollow needle under a blue plastic catheter, tapered on the sharp end and with two ports on the other. I replaced it in the set and picked up a one-and-a-half inch needle and secured it to the top of my lidocaine syringe.

"Now you're going to feel some poking," I explained.

I tried not to think of my isolation in this prairie hospital. In London, I had senior physicians, junior doctors, technicians, and paramedics. I had X-ray labs and ultrasound and CT scanners. I was now in rural Texas, fifty miles from a proper X-ray machine, in an old ER at three in the morning, about to place an internal jugular line in a drug addict, with no backup whatsoever. I let a bubble of panic gather strength, waited a minute, then squashed it. *Please let this work.*

"Here we go," I announced, trying to sound relaxed.

I held the syringe at forty-five degrees to her neck. I aimed for the skin just to the side of my middle left finger. I stretched the skin further and slid the needle in and pulled back on the plunger, creating suction.

Nothing.

I pulled out completely and applied pressure over the site of the puncture with gauze. I reduced the pressure of my left fingers and took a few deep breaths, not looking at Joe.

"Any luck, Doc?" he asked, cheerfully.

I didn't answer.

I tried again. I pushed the needle in about half an inch and pulled back. Nothing. I waited, then tried again.

Nothing.

I could sense Joe getting up impatiently. I kept up the negative pressure in the syringe and pulled back fractionally.

Still nothing.

"Doc Becker *always* gets it in the groin! In five minutes!" he repeated.

I pulled out a little more and watched. Joe walked out. I pulled out even more, perilously close to the surface. Suddenly, a thread of blood shot into the syringe and curled. I stopped and whooped.

"Ben! We're in! Give me the guide wire!"

I held the needle in place and gently disconnected the syringe. Blood welled up and rippled down her neck. I slowly advanced a soft guide wire through the needle. It went in easily and blood stopped pouring out. Joe reappeared.

"You got in?"

"Yeah."

"In the neck?"

"Yeah."

"How do you know you're not in the artery?"

"Because the blood wasn't shooting out under pressure when I pulled off the syringe," I answered smoothly, removing the needle over the guide wire and exchanging it with the blue catheter.

Once the catheter was in all the way, I removed the wire and blood dripped out the end of the catheter. I held it up for Joe. He looked crestfallen.

"Here! Now you can get your blood samples before we start fluids. Then we need an X-ray to confirm position."

I stitched the catheter into place, anchoring its flange, a side flap, to the skin.

"This shouldn't hurt," I explained to Tricia. "I'm stitching the cathe-ter to the skin that I just numbed up."

To my surprise, Tricia had dozed off. She woke with a start.

"Did you get in?" she asked.

"Yes."

"Whoa! You must be good! I've tried that one for *years*, couldn't *ever* get it!"

I shuddered at the thought of her standing in front of a mirror, stab-bing her neck.

"Didn't feel a thing. Good job, Doc!"

Joe collected his samples and left silently. Ben cleaned her neck, removing the towels and wiping off the excess iodine with alcohol. I trimmed the stitches and surveyed the results with satisfaction.

"I just thought of something. During my certification exam in Glasgow, I had to look at the back of a patient's eye. I found something there that *proved* she had bacterial endocarditis. I'm going to look for that now. Ben, give me the ophthalmoscope!"

Ben looked flustered.

"Doc, it's attached to the wall. Won't come that far."

We moved the bed until Tricia was just underneath the wall-mounted instrument. I removed it from the socket and explained.

"This is an instrument to look at the inside of your eye. I'm going to look inside at the blood vessels and the inner lining of the eye, called the retina. I'm going to shine a very bright light and I'm going to come very close to your face."

I remembered that clinical exam in Glasgow. My tight-lipped examiner had asked me to look at the retina on the right side. I had been sure that I would find something significant. I had looked and looked, but had found nothing.

"See anything interesting?" he had asked.

"Nothing! It's totally normal!" I admitted.

Then he had smiled faintly and hissed, "Now examine the *other* side."

And there it was: The first Roth spot I had ever seen. A big, red, evil cherry, a tangle of infected and swollen blood vessels. It was a reliable sign of bacterial endocarditis, and I had made the diagnosis. I smiled at the memory and drew near.

It was there! Smaller, for sure, but there it was *right there!* A red spot, in the center of the retina, a mangled wreck of vicious bacteria and fragile blood vessels. I straightened up.

"She's definitely got endocarditis. I need to send her to Abilene. She needs to be in an ICU. This is serious."

Ben turned to me ruefully.

"Doc, hate to break it to you. You going to have a hard time getting her up there."

"Why?"

He hesitated, and Tricia spoke up.

"Because I'm a frequent flyer and I do drugs and I sell sex and they treat me like shit because of it."

Ben shrugged. I was confident. There was a Roth spot! You can't argue with a Roth spot!

"I'm going to call anyway. You need to be transferred."

Joe returned with the preliminary results.

"She's got a high white count, nineteen thousand. Sed rate's cooking, but looks pretty high. Something's going on."

I went to the small office and called the ER physician, Dr. Lockwood, in Abilene. He was adamant.

"Hell no! We can't accept her! Tricia White, aka White Trash! No, no, no! You're not dumping her on us again!"

"But she's got endocarditis!"

"How do you know? Are her blood cultures positive?"

"We just drew them. They won't be back for forty-eight hours."

"Then call us after forty-eight hours!"

"But she's got a Roth spot and a high white count," I further explained.

"How high?"

"Nineteen thousand."

"Well, that's high, I'll give you that. But our cutoff is twenty. Just keep her, hit her with lots of antibiotics, she'll be fine."

"She needs an echo to look for bacterial vegetations growing on her heart valves."

"You're still going to give her antibiotics. Just start the antibiotics and sit tight. Good luck!"

I had the same results with the ERs in San Angelo and Brownwood. I stepped out wearily. Tricia called out.

"I heard it all. They'll never take me again. Said so last time."

"We need to give you antibiotics by vein for several days. I'm writing your admission orders."

"I'll be admitted under you?"

"Yes."

Ben stepped forward and asked, "Any family with you?"

"Bobby Joe's outside. Bobby Joe Patterson. He's my friend. Put his name down."

Ben looked away and shook his head.

"The whore and the gay guy," he muttered.

I burst out.

"What *is* it with all of you? What's your problem with gays?"

Ben looked at me, shocked. He leaned back against the counter, astonished.

"You like *gays*?" he asked.

"Gays are the same as everyone else," I said. "I have gay friends and straight friends and I like them all, they're *good* people, okay? It's okay to be straight and it's okay to be gay! *Okay?*"

"Okay, Doc, okay!"

I had surprised myself. Normally, I stayed out of these discussions. I didn't want any controversy. I needed the support of this town to get my green card, and I sincerely respected the people. They were honest and generous and welcoming, and I didn't want to reprimand them while asking them a favor. I remembered snapping at Anjali and making her cry. *I don't usually burst out like this. It must be the lack of sleep,* I reasoned, *and maybe the investigation.* Ben cleared his throat.

"Nothing against them. It's just plain *wrong*, that's all."

"No, there's nothing *wrong* with being gay!" I snapped.

Tricia swung around, the central line hanging from her neck.

"Bobby Joe's a good guy," she said. "You better not say a word against him."

Ben retreated and cleared the tabletop angrily. He threw the spent materials in the trashcan and kicked it. He slammed the clipboard down and completed the paperwork, seething.

"Sign here," he ordered.

He noted the tattoos of armadillos on her forearm and sneered, "Tattoos! The common man's contribution to the fine arts!"

I looked up.

"Did you ever watch *MASH*?" I asked. "Guy called Winchester said that."

"I've seen *MASH*," Ben said. "I liked it. I remember Winchester. Was he Simon Winchester?"

"Don't know," I said.

"Anyhow, turned out he was gay in real life. Came out later on."

"So what? There was someone from *Star Trek* too, who came out later on. What's your point?" I asked.

Ben didn't wait for an answer. He reached for a folder and peeled out a form.

"This is the consent for treatment form and it says the patient is *okay with staying in Hotspur and not being transferred out.* You want her to sign it, Doc?"

I recognized the sharpness in his voice and let it drop. I was so tired.

———

I reached home and slept for two hours. I ate breakfast, feeling aggrieved at the world for doubting my intentions, for humiliating me with an investigation, for refusing to accept my patient, for my lack of sleep, for refusing me a green card, and for the generic taste of my pancakes and syrup. I ignored the girls. I thought back about Sparky and Esperanza, and felt reasonably sure that I *had* obtained the consent form. I tried to picture the form but couldn't. I didn't remember seeing Sparky's signature on it, but I might have signed it before he had, or maybe Esperanza had signed the form. Why couldn't I remember? Was I doubting myself? Life was awful. I drank two cups of coffee and pushed away from the table and glared at my children.

"That was a good Akbar-Birbal story last night before bed," Priya said, encouragingly.

Anjali nodded.

"Will you tell it again tonight?" Priya asked.

"Sure, why not. We all want fairness and justice."

Priya soaked her pancake with syrup. She looked up sweetly and shrugged. Her response surprised me.

"It's just a *story*, Dad. *Make up a story* if you want, a new story."

———

We had a clinic chart on Sparky and I reviewed it as soon as I reached the office.

"You may have a ten-thirty, Dr. Mathur. But she didn't confirm," Kendra said.

"No problem. Let me see Esperanza's chart as well."

"She doesn't have a clinic chart. She's never been seen by us."

"Do you think she was Hispanic?"

"Oh yes, she was Hispanic all right!"

"So she was probably Catholic. Is there any other Catholic church here, other than Sacred Heart?"

"Nope. Only Catholic Church in town's Sacred Heart. Small church. We got just a handful of Catholics in town."

I called the church. They had heard of Esperanza, but no one knew her well. They knew nothing of her family. No good friends, only acquaintances. She had not attended services regularly and never volunteered. She had kept to herself, and not attended social events organized by the church. The pastor was unavailable, but they assured me that he would not have much to add. I hung up reluctantly. The brief optimism of the morning had been snuffed out.

Karl appeared in the door. He did not waste time with formalities.

"Hey, man, you're in some deep shit!"

He didn't sound upset.

"I guess."

"You know this is serious business, right?"

"Yes."

"Ah guaran-damn-tee you, this is serious, man! You could lose your license!"

He was chortling.

"Adios to them green cards!"

I flinched.

"Don't remind me. I'm trying to focus on the chart."

"Hey, yeah, spend some time with the chart. You may need to *buff it up* a little! Heard you can make up stories!"

He winked and withdrew. Was he suggesting I *add* something to the chart? Should I write something down, then backdate it, and use it to exonerate myself? I felt a wave of exhilaration. *I could end all this, right now.* This nightmare would be over. I reviewed the chart again and looked for a blank space in the record. I mentally prepared what I would write. Something bland, not too pointed, but sufficient. The word *vindicated* popped up. I was going to be safe.

As I continued to review the chart, I felt resentful. I had done nothing wrong. I had explained everything to Sparky. I had offered to send him to Abilene and to San Angelo. He had refused. I remembered that I had offered to call MD Anderson Cancer Center, where I had done part of my training. He had refused. As those memories returned, I felt reassured.

I thought again about adding to the chart, maybe something bland like *the patient was advised of his transfer options but declined,* or *The patient insists on being treated here only.* I thought about the options. Yes, I could probably get away with it. It had to sound genuine, in bad handwriting so the investigator would have to squint and might even miss it on the first read. I looked around for a pen. There was one right there. I paused. *The pen is right there?* There were never any pens just lying around this area. I thought again. I thumbed through the chart. *There was a blank page there*, in the right place. Should I write something? Something bland, but helpful? Or just go all out and write a detailed note saying I had explained everything to him at length? *What had really happened that morning?* I had tried to save my tie, *that* I was sure of. I had done the admission paperwork. I had *probably* signed the form. Sparky had *probably* signed the form. Esperanza would bear me out, of course. It was going to work out. I quashed any thoughts of buffing. I had done nothing wrong, and the facts would bear me out. The convenient blank page and the available pen be damned! I slammed the chart shut and returned it to Heather.

"Here! Seal this chart! It's Sparky's. We may need it for the investigation."

Karl sipped his coffee thoughtfully and turned the pages of *Big Game Hunter*.

My ten-thirty never showed up. I went down to check on Tricia. She looked better, having rested and cleaned up. Her eyes shone and she sat up straight. She smiled sweetly and waved as I walked in. I checked her vitals. The fever was down. She had received her first dose of vancomycin and gentamicin. I noticed Nelda Smalley, the head nurse, in the corner. She was a sincere woman with a mass of curly hair tied up in a ribbon.

"Nelda, we need to draw blood to check the gentamicin levels."

"May I draw it from her central line, Doctor?"

"Sure. I don't think you can get it anywhere else."

I examined Tricia again. Her heart rate had slowed down and I heard, for the first time, a soft murmur, a faint hiss with each contraction, as blood regurgitated back into the smaller chamber.

"You have a soft systolic murmur, Tricia."

"Is that good or bad?" she asked.

"It may mean that there is some damage to the heart valve. It means the blood flow around the valve is now kind of turbulent. Whenever the large chamber squeezes blood, some of it goes backward, back to the smaller chamber, instead of moving forward."

"Will it get better?"

Nelda interrupted, "You will only get better if you renounce your evil ways, sister! Carrying on with the men and injecting yourself is evil, *bound* to bring punishment. Your evil heart has been punished!"

Tricia seized Nelda's hand.

"I ain't evil, sister!"

"What you do with men is evil!"

"I just keep myself happy, and anyone who comes to me, I keep them happy. I'm in the business of pleasure."

I had not expected this conversation.

Nelda shook her head, lips pursed, as she changed the pillow cover. There was silence for a few minutes. She gathered the bed sheets, then said, "Bless you! You've been sweating with the fever!"

Tricia glared at her, still angry.

"I ain't evil!"

"We're all sinners, sister. You, just more so. You must repent and change your ways!"

She picked up the sheets and the pillow cover and placed them on the breakfast tray. She turned to me.

"May I be of any further assistance to you?" she asked sweetly.

"No, thank you."

Nelda sprayed the room with air freshener and sailed out.

"They all hate me," Tricia whispered.

"Maybe they're afraid of you," I responded.

"I know a lot. I could get them into trouble."

"No one wants trouble."

She looked up slyly.

"I heard *you're* in trouble."

I stopped and turned.

"Who told you that?"

"Everyone knows. Why're you in trouble? You a child molester or something?"

I looked at her. She was calm and plainly curious. I swallowed.

"Actually, the board is investigating me because one of my patients died and they want to make sure that I offered to transfer him to a bigger hospital and didn't just keep him here."

"You tried to transfer me! You tried for me!"

"Tell that to the board."

"I liked how you spoke up for Bobby Joe and gays."

"You're welcome."

"But don't keep saying that. This is Hotspur, this ain't Austin."

"I know."

"Can I go out and smoke?" she asked.

"No."

"I figured you would say that."

As I left the room, she sat up and dropped one leg over the side of the bed. She smiled wickedly.

"Are you interested in me?"

"What?"

"Are you interested in me?"

"No!"

"You looked at me kinda funny."

I put her chart down and choked my irritation.

"You're an interesting patient. You're full of clues. You're tattooed all over. You've got rashes and lumps and splintered nails and red palms and all sorts of medical clues. You're interesting—from a medical point of view."

She liked that. She pulled her leg back up on the bed and pulled up the sheets and covered herself to the neck.

"I'm interesting! Good. You don't think, like, she can't be a real slut, she got no boobs?"

"No!"

"I know I got no boobs! But I got good *hands!*"

She held them up like fans. They were small hands with sharp fingers.

"I can massage *real* good!"

I smiled, not knowing what to say.

"You know what the trick is? Start with the feet and just work up, Doc! Work up, slowly!"

I had nothing to say.

"Men just want to be happy."

"Seems reasonable."

"Men're hunters. Every man hunts. Hunts for what makes him happy!"

"I guess so."

"What makes you happy, Doc?"

"Getting the investigation off my back would make me happy."

I headed out of her room.

"I'll do a little digging about you, mister!" Tricia called out.

I had a meeting with the investigator in John's office. The

investigator sat with me, facing John, and turning dramatically to ask me questions.

"What I don't get is, where *is* she? I mean, all we need to wrap this up is to talk to the wife. Where *is* she?" he wondered.

I shrugged helplessly.

"No offense, but I want you gone as well. Lots of rumors making the rounds. I've called her church and they don't know. I've sent the police to her neighborhood and the house is all boarded up with no forwarding address. The neighbors have no clue and there are no friends or family," I said.

"You check with the post office?" the investigator asked. "Any forwarding address for the mail?"

"I did that," John responded, "but I got nothing. There's no forwarding address. I spoke to Teegarten, Sparky's attorney, the guy who wrote his will and all. Nothing."

"Doc, you got anything you want to say? Any thoughts?"

"Have you double-checked all the hospital records? Could the missing form have been misfiled? It might be in some other patient's records," I said.

"Double-checked and triple-checked. You don't have too many admissions so it wasn't difficult!"

"I guess that's one good thing about having few admissions," John muttered.

The investigator leaned forward and turned to me.

"Doc, I'm going to have to pursue this further. We've hit a dead end. You may have to come to Austin for a hearing in front of a panel, and you may want to bring your own lawyer."

My mouth and tongue started to feel dry. I tried to speak calmly. *I can't afford a lawyer! And I could lose my medical license, my job, and even our green cards!*

"I understand. When might this be?"

"In a couple of weeks. I'm going to have the hospital charts examined by a specialist to see if some papers have been removed, if there are any fresh ink marks, and so forth. I also made a copy of the clinic chart a couple of days ago, and I intend to make another copy before I leave. Just to make sure there haven't been any *changes*. Like some new lines or paragraphs that weren't there before."

He looked at me unblinkingly.

"You know it's a criminal offense to tamper with a chart that's under investigation? Board takes a pretty dim view of a doctor who tries to tamper with the evidence."

"I understand."

My mind flashed back to the chart, the blank page, and the pen. *Had it been a trap?*

"You haven't done something foolish like that, have you?"

I looked back at him just as blankly. *It had been a trap!*

"Why would I?"

"Doctors call it *buffing the chart.*"

"Never crossed my mind," I lied.

———

I reached home early and we ate dinner at five thirty. Maya had made my favorite dish, a lamb stew with onions and mushrooms. We set the table together and toasted thick bread called naan, and buttered it while it was still warm. We scooped up the stew with triangles of naan, and Priya gave us a detailed account of the day's events. She noticed me yawn.

"Dad's sleepy today because he didn't sleep last night," she said.

"Why?" Anjali asked.

"Because he had a patient to see in the hospital."

"Why night?" Anjali wondered.

"People get sick at all times, darling. There isn't a fixed time," Maya explained

"Will you tell us another story tonight?" Priya asked.

"Dad needs to sleep early tonight. Maybe he could tell you a story tomorrow night," Maya said.

The girls scowled.

"He's *always* busy!" they complained.

"By the way, one of your patients called," Maya said.

"Called here? At home?"

"Yes. You know they feel free to call at home here, nothing new about that. She said her name was Trish."

"*Trish?*"

"She left you a number to call. She also said something about wanting you to allow her to smoke."

"Oh, it's Patricia White. That's the patient I saw last night—this morning."

"I hear she's a drug addict and a prostitute," Maya whispered. The girls looked up, suddenly inquisitive. Maya ignored them.

"That's true. I'm treating her for endocarditis, a serious heart infection."

"Does she have AIDS?"

The girls looked puzzled, but we offered no answers.

"I've checked her, and she does not. I can't discuss her medical details."

"I'm worried about you, sticking all sorts of needles into drug addicts. What if you were to stick yourself? You could get AIDS from a needle stick! Remember what happened to Mike Anglesby in Houston?"

I shuddered. Mike Anglesby had been a fellow resident in Houston. He had contracted AIDS three years after a needle-stick injury, and was in and out of ICU all the time with life-threatening infections.

"I remember. I'll be careful."

I looked at the number. I did not recognize the area code, 907. I was puzzled. I thought about discarding it. *Maybe her parole officer, she needs me to explain her absence.* I helped clean up after dinner and decided to make the call. I called from the kitchen after Maya had taken the girls to their room. The phone rang and rang and no one picked up. I hung up. I was puzzled: why would Tricia call me at home to give me a number no one answered? I scanned the Texas area codes in the phone book, but couldn't find it. I checked the number. It had rung somewhere, I reasoned, so it must be a real number. *Where was it?* I changed and came back. The second time round, someone picked up the phone.

"Faith Haven of Hope."

"Oh, hello. My name is Dr. Mathur. I'm calling from Hotspur, Texas. Where is this, please?"

"This is Faith Haven of Hope."

"Yes, but what are you? I mean, what sort of business are you?"

"We are a faith-based private rehab center."

"A rehab center? I got your number from a patient of mine. She may have been at your center."

"Perhaps, doctor. We can't disclose any information about our clients. Is there anything I can help you with?"

"Where are you located?"

"Just outside Fairbanks."

"Fairbanks, Alaska?"

"Yes, doctor. Anything else?"

"I don't know. I don't think so."

"Thank you for calling Faith Haven of Hope."

I hung up and went to bed. Before dozing off, I was struck by a sudden thought. I sat up and dialed again.

"Faith Haven of Hope? Do you have a patient there by the name of Esperanza Cummins or Esperanza Palacios? Her maiden name was Palacios."

"We can't disclose that over the phone."

"I understand, but I'm her doctor. I need to discuss an urgent medical matter with her. Is she there?"

There was a pause.

"What was your name?"

"Dr. Mathur. In Hotspur, Texas."

"We do have a patient from Texas. Please wait while I place you on hold. I need to confirm with the nurse and administrator."

I held on, not daring to breathe. I waited and waited. Finally, she returned.

"She is here, Doctor. Would you like me to connect you?"

I slumped and exhaled.

"Yes, *please.*"

CHAPTER SIXTEEN

Closing In

I called the hospital and left messages for John Abbott, and told Francisca about my conversation with Esperanza. I was sure the news would soon be all over Hotspur. I helped myself to fried eggs and tomatoes, slathered mashed avocado over toast, and sprinkled red pepper flakes over it. Priya and Anjali watched me and smiled knowingly at each other. Anjali soaked her waffle with syrup and ate mightily, leaving brown smears on her nose and cheeks. Priya did the same, but with more élan. I was jubilant. I only stopped thinking about the phone call when Maya questioned me.

"You do remember that Anjali has an appointment today?" Maya asked.

"She does?" I answered, cautiously.

"Uh-huh. With Dr. Argyle, the ENT specialist, in Abilene. About her hearing. You said you would come with us."

"Of course! I had planned on it. I just forgot the exact date. I did tell Karl and the office staff that I would be away."

"What about being on call?" Maya asked.

"Yes, I'm on call, but Karl agreed to cover me."

"Good. We have an appointment at ten, so we should probably leave by eight thirty. Takes an hour to get to Abilene and then there's always paperwork."

"Sounds good. Let me just call the hospital and remind them that I'll be away for the morning. My cell phone's discharged and actually I don't even know where it is."

"You should *always* have your phone. How can you be a doctor without a phone?"

"I think I was charging it at the nurses' station in the hospital. Maybe I left it there. I've given them your number. If I can't find my phone, I'll give them Dr. Argyle's office number as well. We aren't going anywhere else, are we?"

"Well, I thought we might eat at Olive Garden afterwards. Anjali likes it, and I like the minestrone soup they have. But don't give them Dr. Argyle's number. That just doesn't sound appropriate."

"I'll think about it. We may have to keep it a little quick because I have to get back here."

Maya started to say something, then checked herself. She stood up and gathered the plates.

"Let's go together. Anjali and I can wait outside while you pick up your phone. Then we can head off to Abilene."

I called the hospital and checked on Tricia. I thanked her warmly. She felt better and had eaten everything on her breakfast tray. She again asked for permission to smoke in her room, which I denied. She told me that the night staff had been irritated with her as she kept calling them for snacks. She had watched TV until two in the morning and the day staff protested. The day shift head nurse, Nelda Smalley, was in the room when I called, and she took the phone.

"Doctor, if she has the strength to watch TV till *two*, she can go *home*, that's what *I* say," she protested loudly, "but what do *I* know, *I'm* just a nurse. *I'm* not the doctor."

"Well, she is getting better, so maybe soon. How about the blood culture results from Abilene? Did we get them back?"

"No, Doctor. I will call them at nine, they open at eight thirty."

"Thank you. If you need me this morning, I will be at Dr. Argyle's office in Abilene. I'm taking Anjali for a checkup."

"Yes, I knew that. My aunt told me me you were taking Anjali there today."

Well, of course Nelda knew. Miss Rasmussen, Nelda's aunt, lived across the street from us.

"I got Dr. Argyle's number on my Rolodex," Nelda continued. "You'll like him, but he's kind of stern."

"Call me there if you need me. Oh, one other thing. Did I leave my cell phone there?"

"There's a little Nokia no one's claimed sitting here at the nurses' desk. Silver clamshell type."

"That's it! Great, I'll come by and pick it up. Just leave it right there."

I called the hospital and gave Francisca Sophia the number in Alaska

again. I asked her to give the number to Officer Torres, the board investigator, as soon as possible. I toyed with the idea of calling Officer Torres myself, then dismissed it as too forward. I reassured myself that the
matter would soon be wrapped up.

———————————

Twenty minutes later, Maya, Anjali, and I pulled up in front of the
hospital. Ben Grimes, the ER nurse, was there. He rushed forward as I
stepped out.

"Doc, Nurse Smalley's been trying to reach you! She wants you in
one-o-one ASAP! Your patient's had a severe allergic reaction!"

I gave Maya the keys and asked her to wait, and rushed inside, past
the pink ladies as they were setting up, past Joe in the lab, and through
the nurses' station to Tricia's room. I burst in and stopped.

Nurse Smalley was disconnecting tubing from Tricia's neck, and
two young new nurses, Meleigh and Vanessa, were assisting her as she
injected a little heparin to prevent the line from clotting. A bag of saline
and a smaller bag of vancomycin lay discarded on the floor, under a
tangle of plastic IV tubing. Tricia sat up in bed, her knees bent and her
arms curled around them. She looked angry and ignored everyone as
she watched television with determination. The resuscitation cart from
the ER had been pulled into the room, and EKG leads snaked out from
under Tricia's gown. The monitor showed a regular heart rate of eighty
per minute and a blood pressure of one hundred ten by seventy, both of
which were satisfactory.

"What happened?" I asked.

"What happened? I'll *tell* you what happened, Doctor. This little
lady had a severe allergic reaction to your antibiotic! Lucky for her I was
in the room when it happened, otherwise who knows what might have
happened to her!"

"She had an allergic reaction? To vancomycin?" I repeated.

"That's right. Face went red as a tomato, all blotchy, couldn't breathe,
everything!" Nurse Smalley answered. "If I hadn't been here, oh, I don't
even want to think about it! *Lord* have mercy!"

She shook her head and shivered. Nurse Smalley was a short lady
with an abundance of curly blonde hair that she kept pinned underneath a small, white nurse's hat. She wore half-moon glasses and threw
her head back repeatedly as she peered at Tricia's neck.

"I reckon I should take this line out now," she observed. "We can always give antibiotics by mouth."

"No, don't do that!" I said. "That was a difficult line and she doesn't have any other sites. Don't take it out!"

Nurse Smalley looked disappointed and stared at me down the bridge of her nose.

"She had an allergic reaction to vancomycin, Doctor! She can't have that again!"

"Look, there's something wrong. This is her third day on vanco! How could she develop an allergy on day three? If she had a true allergy, it would have developed right away, in minutes after the first dose!"

"Well, all I can say is, it was a severe allergic reaction! But what do *I* know, *I'm* only a nurse, not a doctor!" she said, shaking her head and rolling her eyes.

Meleigh and Vanessa smirked.

I sighed, then resumed," Look, let me ask you this. Her vanco should have been given at three a.m., because it's every twelve hours, three a.m. and three p.m. Why was she getting it now, at eight o'clock?"

"The night shift was busy, Doctor! They didn't get around to it!"

"That's my point. I think they gave it late and so they were in a hurry to finish it. Vanco can cause a reaction with redness and flushing when given too fast. It's called red man syndrome."

"Never heard of such a thing," Nurse Smalley said.

Meleigh and Vanessa rolled their eyes.

"I've seen this reaction to vancomycin before, and it's simply related to the rate at which the antibiotic is dripped into the patient. If given too fast, it can cause that kind of reaction."

Nurse Smalley jammed her hands onto her hips and raised her voice. "We can't take that kind of chance, Doc!"

"Well, the blood culture results are here now and the bacteria are resistant to most of the antibiotics we have, but they are sensitive to vancomycin. She really needs it. Maybe she's not really allergic to vanco. Maybe she just had that reaction because vanco was given too fast."

Nurse Smalley stood silently and shook her head in disbelief. Meleigh and Vanessa looked incredulous. The phone rang and they ignored it.

"Sir, I *personally* saw the woman collapse. She was a goner, I thought. And when we got her back, she looked like death warmed up. I don't agree. You should *not* give that woman vancomycin!"

There was a knock on the door and Officer Torres stepped in.

"Doc, there's a lady, I believe it's your wife, at the nurses' station. She's asking how long you're going to be, because you have an appointment in Abilene."

"Thanks, Officer. Would you please tell her it's going to take fifteen minutes, I'll call her, she can wait in the clinic upstairs."

Officer Torres nodded and paused.

"Okay. Everything all right here?"

"No," Nurse Smalley burst out. "No, it's not. This patient almost died from an allergic reaction and her doctor wants me to give her the same medicine again. I can't! I can't risk losing my license!"

Officer Torres stepped in and looked at me sternly.

"Let me talk to the patient," I said.

I turned to Tricia. She didn't look up but held a finger to her lips.

"Luciano's gonna get it!"

I sat down next to her and looked at the television screen. Three gangsters were sitting at a bar, laughing and slapping each other on the back, then two walked away. Tricia clicked her tongue in warning

"Luciano's gonna get it!" she repeated.

A shadowy character suddenly appeared and threw a rope around Luciano's neck and pulled violently. Luciano thrashed around and clawed at his neck. His face turned red and ballooned grotesquely. He collapsed in a heap. The assassin spat on him. Tricia sighed and pressed the mute button.

"That's what she looked like!" Nurse Smalley exclaimed.

"Did they tell you what happened?" Tricia asked, wearily.

"Yes."

"I almost died!"

"Give me the details."

Tricia crossed her legs and looked at the ceiling and thought back. She looked like a college student, a wisp of a girl with slicked-back hair, an earnest face, bright eyes and slender limbs, and fresh makeup over the sites of needle-sticks and tattoos.

"I felt this *heat* come on all over me. I felt just real warm and my face turned real red. The nurse said, 'Oh my, Tricia, what's wrong?' and I said, 'Don't know what's happening.' My voice sounded strange so she checked me good and said, 'Whoa, you're real sick. Low blood pressure.' She checked both arms and legs. She laid me down real flat and said, 'Stay like that,' and she ran and got another bag of—something and squeezed that sucker into me. She sat and watched me lying flat in bed."

"Did your throat swell up?"

"Nope."

"Did your lips swell up?"

"Nope."

"Did you have difficulty breathing?"

"Just felt real hot."

"Was your face red? Your body, did it turn red?"

"I guess. Wasn't looking in the mirror."

"But did your body turn red? Did you see your arms? Did they turn red?"

"Think so. Maybe."

"You can't be sure?"

"Well, *maybe* I was red all over."

"Why? What were you doing? You were lying here in bed, having an attack of something, surely you noticed what your skin looked like?"

She glared back and waved at the TV.

"*The Mafia Murders* was on!" she exclaimed, and turned the sound back on.

"Tricia! Stop that! I really need to figure out if you had a severe allergic reaction or not!"

She sighed and turned the TV off.

"Okay."

"Any itching?"

"Little bit. Afterward."

"Any difficulty swallowing?"

"Nope."

"So there was no rash on your face or body, no hives, no swelling of the throat and no difficulty breathing or swallowing?"

"Look, I think I had a rash but that's all. Okay, felt weird, too. That's it."

She returned to the TV. I was puzzled. I stepped outside with Nurse Smalley and Officer Torres. Nurse Smalley was jubilant.

"Well? You believe me now?" she crowed.

"Well, I agree she had a reaction. I think it was the red man syndrome."

"What's that?" Officer Torres said.

"When vancomycin is given too fast, it can sometimes cause the release of histamine and so you get a red rash all over the body. It's usually pretty bad and affects the upper half of the body. But it's not a true allergy. All we have to do is give the vancomycin slowly, and she should be fine."

Nurse Smalley was not pleased. She shook her head and stepped back, feet apart, hands on hips. Meleigh and Vanessa came and stood behind her.

"You're really going to do this?" she asked.

"What?"

"Give her vanco."

"It's my decision," I said.

Officer Torres followed the exchanges as if he was a spectator at a tennis match.

"I don't believe it! After what I said, you still want her to have vancomycin?" she asked.

"It wasn't a true allergy."

"And what if it was?"

"I've seen this reaction before."

"You can never be a hundred percent sure."

"True, but I'm reasonably sure."

"Reasonably?"

"That's what I said. *Reasonably.*"

"I say it was a severe allergy. I won't give it again."

She turned away and crossed her arms. Officer Torres watched me. Everyone was listening. I hesitated, knowing that the length of my pause was being monitored. I flirted with the idea of abandoning the effort. *I could rush off to Abilene and let them deal with it. Could she survive without the vancomycin? Should I switch to something else that might or might not work? What if I were wrong? If Tricia collapsed, would that cost me my license? My green card? My family's green cards?* Nurse Smalley had already put me on notice.

"I've seen this happen before," I repeated, trying hard to keep my voice steady. "And I'm pretty sure it's the red man syndrome. Her symptoms don't suggest a true allergy to vanco. There was nothing to suggest a severe reaction such as anaphylaxis. She had tolerated it well so far."

Nurse Smalley shook her head in dismay and continued to look away.

"I don't think so. But *I'm* just a nurse, *I'm* not the doctor. I still believe I saw a severe allergic reaction."

"It can be hard to tell the two things apart."

Meleigh and Vanessa looked extremely skeptical.

"So you want to take a chance? Chance on her life? *Her life?*"

Officer Torres looked grim. I became determined. *The State is investigating me, the nurses are doubting me, someone's setting traps for me, and I'm sick of it!*

"I will give the vanco myself. In fact, I will even draw it up myself, mix it myself, and give it IV myself. *Okay?*"

Nurse Smalley glared back defiantly. Meleigh and Vanessa stiffened.

I went on, angrily.

"*I* will sit in the room. *I* will wait right there and watch her and if there is any sign of anaphylaxis or severe allergy, *I* will stop the vancomycin and give her adrenaline."

The three nurses didn't say anything.

"Get me the crash cart. Move it into the room. And call the paramedics. Get me a seven French ET tube, just in case I need to intubate her. Don't open the tube, just have it ready. I need the Mackintosh forceps, just in case she crashes. And get the respiratory tech in the room, if she's still here. Someone tell my wife we're delayed another ten minutes."

Nurse Smalley left reluctantly to retrieve the crash cart from the ER. She mumbled and shook her head. Meleigh and Vanessa crossed their arms and stepped back, to show solidarity with Nurse Smalley. I took a deep breath and ordered sternly.

"You two, come with me. Get me fifty mg of Benadryl IV and ten cc of epi. I want the one in ten thousand strength, *not* the one in a thousand. And a bag of normal saline, five hundred ml. *Now!*"

I marched back to Tricia's room and explained the plan to her.

"I really think you'll be safe. I will stand right here and watch you. If you feel your throat swell up or any difficulty breathing, say so right away or just wave your hand. I will give you the adrenaline and the Benadryl. You understand?"

"Uh-huh," Tricia said, riveted to *The Mafia Murders*. There was a high-speed car chase. She didn't understand or care about what I said.

Meleigh stuck her head in the door.

"Dr. Mathur, your wife called to remind you that you have to go to Abilene for your daughter's appointment."

"Tell her I'll be there soon."

Tricia seemed unimpressed by the gravity of the situation. She turned back to the TV and defiantly raised the volume again. I set up the extra bag of saline so that it would flow easily, ready to deliver emergency drugs. I checked the expiration date on the epinephrine and the Benadryl. I primed the epinephrine so it was ready for use instantly. Nurse Smalley reappeared at the door and informed me tersely that the crash cart was ready and the paramedics were on their way.

"Just in case," she announced in a stage whisper. "Just in case she crashes and burns."

To my astonishment, she then came in and stood by my side.

"I still don't agree, Doc, but I've got your back."

Officer Torres appeared at the door. He looked stern and worried.

"Sorry to interrupt, Dr. Mathur, but could you come by and visit with me in the pharmacy for a minute?"

"Actually, no, I can't right now. We are about to start an antibiotic for this lady and I need to be here in the room. But I'll come there as soon as I'm done."

"Okay, then I'll ask you one of my two questions. First, are you sure you want to do this? Seems like you're taking a little risk. Don't let pride get in the way of good judgment."

"I'm reasonably confident."

He shrugged.

"Second, please come to the pharmacy when you're done here."

He looked long and hard around the room, nodded at the nurse, and disappeared. Tricia didn't look at him and reached for a soda.

"You can start now. Commercial break," Tricia announced.

We got to work. Vancomycin was measured, the concentrations were read out loud, and I double-checked. She drew up saline and injected it into the bottle of vancomycin, removed the needle, and shook it vigorously. She used a larger syringe and drew out all the contents and handed me the empty container to verify. I nodded and she proceeded to inject the contents into a plastic bag of saline.

"This time I'll be slow. *Real* slow," Nurse Smalley said.

I watched the drops form and pool in the air trap at the top of the IV tubing.

"Still dripping too fast!" I said.

"Then it's going to take forever!" Nurse Smalley retorted.

"Slow it down," I ordered. "It needs to be half that rate."

We watched and waited. The minutes passed. I grasped the adrenaline and stood up. Tricia raised a finger to her lips. The car chase ended with a pileup and police started shooting from behind their cars. A gangster machine-gunned them, and then was incinerated as his car exploded. A helicopter swooped down and riddled the area and police reinforcements poured in.

The pharmacist, Joshua Blackwell, appeared at the door. He was a small, clean-shaven man with white hair parted in the middle and wore bifocals. He jammed his hands in the pockets of his white coat and rocked as he spoke.

"Investigator wants to talk to you. In the pharmacy. Now!"

We ignored him. We watched, entranced, as the police gradually got the upper hand. They ran up stairwells and shot down at the Mafiosi. The helicopter made another pass and wiped out stragglers. Snipers shot anything that moved. A few more explosions, and mangled bodies were flung around. A single villain appeared with a rocket launcher, but was shot dead by a sniper. There was huge yellow flash, and all the windows blew out.

"How long has it been?" I asked Nurse Smalley abruptly.

She looked startled.

"Five minutes."

"I'll wait another ten or fifteen minutes. I want to be here, just in case."

Joshua had been watching with us. He shrugged, said, "Whatever," and retreated.

Tricia was still mesmerized. She wanted to see if anyone had survived the mayhem. I glanced around her room. A small suitcase lay open near the sink, where cigarette stubs floated in the water; a bottle of hand cream and a compact lay open on the other side. Loose paper lay on the right side; Tricia had been reading while she brushed. I looked back at her. She sat up, her arms wrapped around her knees, her mouth opening and closing, totally engrossed. The intravenous line hovered beside her neck, and she touched it several times to steady it. The monitor showed a steady pulse of seventy per minute, and I was reassured.

I looked at Meleigh and Vanessa. They, too, stood frozen, hypnotized by the screen. A commercial break started. Tricia groaned, touched the mute button, and fell back, looking sullenly at the ceiling. Her heart rate slowed down to sixty-five. For a few minutes, the only sound was that of the monitor.

"Is that bad, when it's slow?" she asked, still looking up at the roof.

"No, that's good. It's good to have a slow heart rate, around fifty or sixty at rest, so long as you feel okay. You're not short of breath or having chest pain?"

"Nope."

"Then it's good that you have a heart rate of sixty-five per minute."

"You think I'll live?"

"I think so."

"One of my friends said I might die or need a heart transplant."

"I don't think so."

She was silent again.

"I've been smoking. In the bathroom."

Nurse Smalley broke in.

"I know that. I've taken your pack."

"I got another."

"Then hand it over," Nurse Smalley demanded.

"Go find it. Bet you can't."

Nurse Smalley snorted and marched off into the bathroom. She entered it and turned the light on and shrieked in horror.

"Patricia! You sick, sick child!"

Tricia smiled with satisfaction as the nurse groaned and sprayed and flushed repeatedly.

"Three-day dump! Saved it for her. For taking my cigarettes."

"Doctor! Do something!" Nurse Smalley protested.

"What can *I* do? *I'm* only a doctor, *I'm* not the nurse," I told her.

Nurse Smalley laughed. I excused myself from the room and sprinted to the pharmacy.

"So there was no problem with Miss Patricia? No reaction to the vancomycin?" Officer Torres asked.

"No, none at all. Why do you ask?"

"Curiosity. Part of my job. You know, sometimes I come looking for A and I find B. Sometimes, B is more interesting than A. Sometimes I find A *and* B *and* C. Just never know."

235

"So what did you find out, Officer?" I asked.

"Well, the lady in Alaska pretty much bore out your story, seems to like you as a doctor, too. Said nice things about you. Says you told them to go to Abilene, but her husband refused. She isn't a hundred percent sure of the form, whether he signed it or not, but she's sure you told her about it and about their options. We missed the deadline, so I still have to file a report in Austin, but I will recommend that they dismiss the matter. And they usually agree with my assessments."

"So I just have to wait and hear from Austin about the final decision?"

"Yep. But there should be no problem."

"So you're done? Leaving soon?"

"Not so fast. When I was talking to Miss Alaska, I asked her how much morphine her husband took, and you know what she said? She said, hardly any. Maybe a little bit at the end."

"So what? Many people do that. They don't want to be sleepy or confused at that time."

"But there is morphine signed out *every four hours* in the log. Every four hours, like clockwork, six milligrams! Seventy-two milligrams in two days! Did you know that?"

"I didn't."

"You ordered it."

"Yes, but I ordered it to be given as needed, not regularly."

"I'm aware of that. But there was morphine taken out of the pharmacy, and the record says it was given to your patient. But his wife says he never took it."

He leaned over and stared balefully into my eyes.

"Doc, this stinks. Someone's stealing morphine from the pharmacy. I aim to find out real soon where it wound up."

"I had nothing to do with it," I said angrily, taking a step back.

"I don't think you do, but I'm checking. Usually is a pharmacist or nurse. Could even be a doctor."

"I have nothing to do with this. This is ridiculous. Investigate all you want. But I have to go. My daughter has an appointment in Abilene."

"No problem, Doc. That'll be all, for now."

The drive to Abilene was uneventful. Initially, Maya was upset about the delay, but, luckily, we still had enough time, and she calmed down. We sped out past rolling landscapes of mesquites and live oaks, wild grasses and cacti, and stretches of rocky land dotted with straggly patches of red and brown turf. There were small water holes in verdant squares surrounded by bushes and stubby cedars and plump cattle, all framed in polygons of barbed wire. A few cars and trucks whizzed by on the other side, and drivers waved as they passed.

Maya was quiet. I knew it was her concern about Anjali's hearing problems. To me, Anjali was a normal child who participated fully in everything. I didn't believe we had a serious problem. I knew that she didn't talk as much as her sister, but I attributed it to Priya's chattering. Anjali always seemed to understand what was said and simply agreed with Priya most of the time. True, she rarely started a conversation, but always seemed animated and involved. I hoped that Maya's concerns would soon be put to rest.

Dr. Argyle was a well-known ear, nose, and throat specialist. His office was just off the freeway. We cruised along the feeder road, then entered a neat parking lot under a sign that said *ENTrance*. We parked and walked in, with Anjali skipping in happily ahead. Upon entering the doctor's office, she was fascinated by the large aquarium in the waiting room and scrambled around it, chasing the fish. She pointed out the castle with a drawbridge and the plastic skull-shaped cave with a pirate. We filled out the paperwork and handed the receptionist our insurance cards. I hinted that I was a doctor. The receptionist smiled knowingly. She was an older lady, a tall brunette in scrubs, with a large hearing aid bulging out her right ear.

"Yes, Dr. Argyle is expecting you. You work in Brownwood, right?"

"No, Hotspur. I work in Hotspur."

"Oh, Hotspur. They still have a hospital there?"

"Yes. That's where I work."

"Oh, I thought it closed years ago."

"We're very much open. We have an active ER and clinic and hospital with in-patients. I've been sending you patients."

"Uh-huh," she nodded blankly and then turned back to her computer screen.

"Do you know how much longer it will be?" I asked.

"Oh, Dr. Argyle usually runs on time. He'll be with you real soon. Have a seat."

Maya looked up expectantly as I returned.

"They say he's on time. Shouldn't be long."

We sat down and looked around. Framed certificates engraved with gold letters spoke of Baylor College of Medicine in Houston and the University of Texas in Austin. Photographs of scuba divers mingled with those of brilliant phosphorescent fish, all signed *A. Argyle* in the corner. I wondered where he might have taken those shots, and when, and whether they were tax-deductible.

Dr. Argyle didn't keep us waiting. He emerged through a corner door in the waiting room. He was impressive. Tall, lean, with slate eyes, black-rimmed glasses, and a mane of white hair. A cautious smile and firm handshake later, we were in an examination room and Maya was filling him in with details of Anjali's delayed hearing. He nodded and reviewed the paperwork we had just filled out. Occasionally, he would hold up a finger for silence and ask a question. He conjured a gleaming fountain pen the size of a cigar and made quick notes.

Abruptly, Dr. Argyle stood up and stood in front of Anjali. He used a flashlight to peer inside her mouth. He inspected intently and nodded, apparently confirming everything he had suspected. Another flourish, and he was at her side, using the otoscope to examine her eardrums. Anjali didn't even whimper, awed by this magician. I watched in dismay. Karl Becker, and now Austin Argyle? How could I possibly compete?

"Dr. Mathur, what did you think?"

"What?"

"What did you think?"

"Of what?"

I saw Maya's irritated expression and bit my lip.

"I'm sorry. I wasn't paying attention. What was the question?"

"What did you think of Anjali's eardrums?"

"What did I think of the eardrums?" I repeated, hollowly.

"Yes, her eardrums. Her *tympanic membranes*. What did you think of her eardrums, Dr. Mathur?"

"I thought they were inflamed."

"When did you last examine her eardrums?"

"About two or three weeks ago."

I was starting to dislike him. I tried to keep the irritation out of my voice.

"It was closer to Halloween, Dr. Argyle," Maya said. "So it must have been at least two months ago."

"Well, the child has a perforation in the right eardrum and the other one is *severely* inflamed," Dr. Argyle said.

"She has a *perforation?* In her eardrum?" I asked, incredulously.

"Indeed she does. Here, let me show you."

He yanked a flat screen forward and touched the menu. Instantly, a picture of the eardrum appeared and he pointed out a small black spot in the upper quadrant of the picture. There was the perforation. Dr. Argyle rapped at it vigorously with his fountain pen.

"There! Do you see it?"

"Yes, I think I do."

"You *think* you do? That is a very clear perforation."

"I see it," I admitted.

"*Textbook* quality. That perforation could be in a textbook!"

My face grew hot.

"Well, I examined her with my hand-held otoscope, and I didn't see it."

Dr. Argyle paused, a disbelieving look on his face.

"Ah. I see."

"After all, I am a gastroenterologist. My specialty involves other openings."

There was another awkward silence. Dr. Argyle froze for a few seconds, incredulous, then shook his head. I looked away, avoiding Maya's gaze. I didn't dare look at Anjali.

"Dr. Mathur?"

The receptionist stood at the door, holding a piece of paper. I was bewildered.

"The nurse at the Hotspur hospital wants to talk with you. Says it's urgent."

"You gave them the number here?" Maya asked. "And you *still* don't have your cell phone?"

"I have my phone but it's dead. It didn't charge for some reason. Remember, I have that very sick patient," I explained. "She has a rare disease."

"Then maybe she should be in Abilene," Dr. Argyle murmured.

"They won't take her. I've been trying to get her to Abilene or Brownwood but they just won't take her."

Dr. Argyle shrugged and sat down. He wrote in the chart. Maya looked away. I stood up and excused myself. I answered in the corridor outside.

"This is Dr. Mathur."

"Hey, Doc! Sorry to bother you!" Nurse Smalley sang out.

"No problem," I lied. "What's up?"

"Well, St. James Hospital just called. Lab says her blood cultures sure are positive! They're saying you're right, she's got endocarditis."

"Really!"

I felt a flush of victory.

"And the head of the medical team wants to speak with you!"

"About what?"

"I guess to apologize and accept the patient."

"Great! What's his name? Did he leave a number?"

"Yep! Done given it to the receptionist, Donna Sue."

"Did they say anything else?"

"Yeah, they asked how you ended up in Hotspur. *His good luck*, I told them."

She laughed and I smiled.

"Well, call me when you're done. Or you can tell Donna Sue, Dr. Argyle's receptionist. Turns out, we're kin!"

The receptionist looked up at the mention of her name and nodded. She handed me a note. I called Dr. DeFord, chief of medical staff at St. James Hospital, the local referral hospital in Abilene.

"Dr. Maythorn?"

"Actually, it's Mathur. Sounds like Martha, you know, George Washington's wife."

"Marthore, Marthore. Yes, got it. Well, I'm Gus DeFord, and I want to tell you that we have reviewed your request to transfer Miss Patricia White. We have decided to accept her to our ICU."

"Great! She really needs to be there."

"I want to apologize for not accepting her right away. The ER called me for advice and I told them not to accept the patient. Fact is, I have never seen a Roth spot in my life. And here you are, diagnosing bacterial endocarditis in the boondocks with an ophthalmoscope and a look at the retina and you find a damn Roth spot!"

"Well, I had seen one before, so I knew to look."

"You've seen one before? Where?"

"In London. During my membership exams, actually."

"In London? What were you doing in London?"

"I trained there. I got my membership, which is the British equivalent of board certification here."

"And what are you doing in Hotspur, for Christ's sake?"

"They offered me a green card."

"That's a good reason. How long do you have to stay there?"

"At least three years."

"And then?"

"I haven't thought about that."

"Let me know. We may have an opening for you."

He rang off. I called the nurses' station in Hotspur and ordered the transfer. I was glowing as I walked back into the examination room. Dr. Argyle did not look up.

"That was Dr. DeFord from St. James Medical Center. They've decided to accept my patient after all. They agree with the diagnosis. The blood cultures came back positive. She definitely has bacterial endocarditis."

I looked around. No one was listening. Dr. Argyle finished writing a prescription, stood up, and handed it to Maya.

"Have Anjali start this *immediately*. Follow up in four weeks!"

"Yes, Dr. Argyle, sir," Maya said politely.

I watched her in astonishment. She was in awe. I thought she would curtsy. Dr. Argyle turned and galloped past me.

He threw me a look of disgust and muttered, "Roth spot!" and added, "but *missed* a perforation on his *own daughter!*"

He stopped at the reception and announced, "No charge!"

And he was gone.

"*Why* did you give the hospital Dr. Argyle's number?" Maya asked, cold fury etched all over her face.

"I was hoping that they would agree to the transfer. I wasn't expecting the cultures to come back positive so soon. That was a real bonus."

"Don't you realize that your daughter has been running around with a hole in one ear and an infection in the other?"

"Of course I do! I was surprised to see the perforation!"

"Because you missed it! Doesn't it bother you at all?"

"Of course it does! But it is a tiny perforation. It will heal up nicely. Yes, yes, I missed it but I haven't been looking at a lot of eardrums in London and Houston. After all, I'm an internist and gastroenterologist."

"You're also her *father*."

"Yes, I know."

"Don't they teach you how to look at eardrums in internal medicine?"

"Yes, but I don't see children. I don't see anyone under eighteen."

"What about the ER?"

"Well, yes, you're right. Over there I have to see everyone. But I would have probably given Anjali an antibiotic as well."

I looked at Anjali. She had wandered back to the aquarium and was watching the clownfish and anemones with great fascination.

"But you hadn't looked at her ears in so long!"

"Yes, true, true. I should have checked them again. I should have started antibiotics sooner."

We drove back in silence after that, our anger suppressing our hunger. I felt ashamed that I had missed Anjali's problems and also a little aggrieved by Dr. Argyle's remarks. I realized how foolish I had been and felt the bitter bile of regret. I looked at Anjali in the rearview mirror. She smiled, then looked outside. How could I have neglected her, I wondered. Anjali sensed the tension and remained silent. Olive Garden was out of the question.

Everyone was looking for me at the hospital. John Abbott grabbed my forearm immediately.

"Doc Sandy! Where in blazes have you been? The investigator's looking for you!"

"Where is he?"

"He's with the pharmacist in the pharmacy room. Nurses' station."

He escorted me there and rapped on the glass window of the door.

"Officer Torres! Here he is!"

Officer Torres was poring over some logbooks. Joshua, the pharmacist, stood behind him, visibly upset. Officer Torres looked up briefly and pointed to the nurses' station. We sat down there and waited. John Abbott looked at the hospital census board and gave a low whistle.

"Whoa! We have six patients!"

"I guess."

"That's great! We used to only have one or two!"

"It's only going to help the hospital if they have insurance," I spoke without thinking.

John looked surprised.

"Since when have you been thinking like that, Doc Sandy?"

"Sorry, it sounds callous," I said, sheepishly.

"Heck, no! I like it! I'm going to find out how many have insurance. You best stay right here, wait on Mr. Torres."

He wrote down the names of the patients and rushed off to his office. I sat and waited. I wondered if he had been able to contact Alaska again, and what Esperanza might or might not have said. *What if she had recanted everything and said I had forced them to stay? How would I prove her wrong then? It would be my word against hers.* I glanced idly at the Post-it notes stuck on the ledge and on the wall. *Karl called, running late. Morris Funeral Home 6254009 Abilene Regional Hospital 9156924000, Poison center 1800 poisons, Dr Mathur home 6254882.*

I looked for something with an Alaska area code but found nothing. I glanced at the trashcan, but decided against rummaging through it. I still felt there was some sort of conspiracy. I pulled Tricia's folder from the rack and looked under *Lab* for the latest entries. *Blood cultures positive, sensitivities to follow. White count coming down, though still elevated. Low albumin levels, probably due to poor nutrition. Tests for syphilis, HIV, hepatitis B and C were negative. Urine cultures were negative.* I looked for and found the consent for treatment form, and read it again, and checked her signature. She *had* consented to stay in Hotspur and get treated here—*there it was*—in black and white. I looked at her medication record. Nothing unusual. She was not on morphine or Demerol, and was not asking for anything for pain either. She was taking methadone, commonly given for recovering drug addicts. Other than complaints about her food and the attitude of the staff, her record was straightforward. I wrote a progress note about my conversation with Dr. DeFord, and ordered the entire chart copied to speed up her transfer. I went to the coffee machine in the break room.

Officer Torres joined me and poured himself some coffee.

"Well, I called the number you gave me again and I spoke to the lady there and she again confirmed what you said. Like I said, we had missed the deadline, so I still have to file the case in Austin."

"You told me that. Do I have to come to Austin?"

"I'm going to recommend that the case be dismissed, pending written confirmation of my discussion with the wife."

"So what do I do?"

"Just be patient."

"Is my license at risk?"

"Nope. Well, technically, yes, because we missed the deadline, so I got to file a report and all, but I don't think it's going anywhere, Doc. You're good."

A wave of relief came over me. I cradled his words silently.

"Will you report this investigation in the monthly newsletter?"

"You mean, will we print your name in the Hall of Shame? In our monthly newsletter we send all the docs in Texas? You bet."

He looked at my crestfallen face and laughed.

"Hey, I'm just messing with you, Doc!"

He thumped me on the back and poured himself some more coffee.

"Naw, you won't be in the Hall of Shame. We only report final actions there, you know, once we make a final determination that there's some kind of serious shortcoming. You know Doc, all the docs in Texas read that list, just to see if any of their friends got in trouble."

"I do look at that list."

"Sure you do. Try to read between the lines. Alcohol, sex, or drugs? If sex, then with whom? A patient? A minor? Just read the punishments and think the worst and you'll be right ninety-nine percent!"

"Is there a lot of it?"

"What, breaking the law? Heck, yeah. You think docs are any different from the rest of us ordinary human beings?"

"We try to be."

"We all hold docs to a high standard, but they're all human. Make mistakes."

"Why? Why do they make mistakes?"

"Well, they have this *image* thing. So they lie. They lie that they're not tired, they lie that they have enough money, they lie that they're like God. Then they take drugs or steal or, you know, take liberties with patients or nurses or others."

"What do you *really* think about doctors?" I asked sarcastically.

"I have a lot of regard for them, Doc. Really, I do. They all try so hard, least most of them do. They all mean well, you know, usually have good intentions."

I had never met any doctor who had been punished, and I felt he was being unfair. We sipped coffee and looked out the door at the nurses' station.

"Hey, tell me, Doc, that patient of yours who died, do you remember if he took a lot of narcotics? I know I've asked you this. Maybe you've had time to think about it."

"What do you mean?"

"Well, he was dying. So did he need a lot of morphine? Or Demerol?"

"Let me think. You know, I can't remember that he did. In fact, I wrote for morphine for him, but I think he declined it."

"If he was in pain why would he decline it?"

"Because he said he was suffering from a personal loss. He said the morphine made him confused and he wanted to keep the memory of his loss, his personal loss. So he declined the morphine a lot of the time. Not all the time, but a lot of the time."

"So he didn't get it every four hours regularly?"

"I don't think so."

He chewed on the edge of the coffee cup.

"So he died in pain?"

"I wasn't here when he died, but the nurses said he died pretty quickly. He had a big cancer near one of the major blood vessels in the chest, and I think it eroded into the aorta. I think he bled internally and died pretty quickly. But that's just my guess, you know; his wife refused an autopsy."

"Yes, I know. *That* form's in the chart."

My face burned and I looked away.

"Well, I checked with the wife and she confirmed everything you said. She said he was dead set against all narcotics, said he had seen what it did to his dad before he died, so he didn't want any part of it."

He leaned forward and pointed at me.

"I know about his son. She told me."

"That was personal."

"Sure. That was right, not to tell me that. But she did."

"So if you knew about his refusing narcotics, why are you asking me so much?"

He grinned.

"Always checking. Seeing if your version fits with the wife's. Heck, she could be lying!"

"How does this have anything to do with his decision to stay here in Hotspur?"

"It doesn't. See, Doc, while investigating, I found that narcotics had been taken out from the pharmacy for your patient. You had written an order for morphine three to four mg every four hours as needed for pain."

"We have already been over that. What—"

"Hang on. You wrote it, that's okay. You wrote it when he was admitted, that's okay. He declined it. That's okay. Problem is, it was issued from the pharmacy and signed out to the patient's account *every four hours!* Nursing notes *don't* say he refused it. Don't clearly say anything."

"So does this mean that this investigation will go on?"

"Yes."

"So I'm still under investigation?"

Officer Torres drained his coffee and wiped his mouth with the back of his hand and looked away.

"Nope, you're okay. I'm satisfied. *You're* clear."

I looked in the same direction as Officer Torres. He was staring at the nurses' station.

"But I need to investigate something else, Doc. There's a *bunch* of morphine missing. And I have a feeling there's a whole lot more that's missing."

"But *I'm* clear?"

He shrugged.

"Yes. Yes, sir, you're clear!"

I didn't hear anything else. I was elated. I was clear. My license was intact. I would not be reported. I could continue to work and get a salary and apply for green cards and citizenship! I rushed out to the nurses' station to call Maya, flushed with relief.

Karl was sitting at the nurses' station and looked at me with amusement.

"Whoa! Looks like you just took a monster dump!"

I grinned.

"It's a big relief."

"You off the hook?"

"Yes."

"Totally?"

"Yes."

"Good for you, man."

Officer Torres appeared and spoke quietly.

"Dr. Becker, may I have a word with you? In the pharmacy?"

I didn't pay attention. I snatched the phone. At the stairwell, Joe stopped me.

"Hey, Doc!"

"Hey, Joe!"

I was surprised to see Joe looking sheepish.

"Doc, I want to thank you."

"Thank me? What for?"

"Well, you know you always been telling us to wear gloves when we draw blood? For blood samples and such?"

"I know that you all don't really like it, because it's harder to feel the veins when you're wearing gloves."

"Right, right. Well, thing is, this here investigator comes in our lab, says he's just a-looking, sits down really polite and starts reading a paper. So we all looked at him and he don't pay us any mind, so we just go about our business. Turns out, he was watching us to see if we was wearing gloves when doing blood draws."

"So it was a trap?"

"Yes! A trap!"

"And were you wearing gloves?"

"Well, thank God it was one of your patients and you had written *Use Gloves* all over the form, so we *had* to. Kind of saved us."

"Hey, that's great!"

Joe hesitated, squirmed, and squeezed his eyes shut, then finally spoke through gritted teeth.

"Guess I just want to say thanks," he whispered.

The he scurried back into the lab.

I walked past the Pink Ladies and wished them well. They asked about Anjali, and I told them about the perforation. They were sympathetic. I stopped at Francisca's desk and thanked her for her help. John was standing there and looked pleased and relieved.

We shook hands and he had me sit down in his office.

"Great news, great news! You're off the hook!"

"Are you sure?"

"Just a technicality left! Letter from Austin!"

"So I shouldn't worry?"

"Not at all. And have I got a surprise for you."

"What?"

"Well, you know the Chamber of Commerce dinner tonight? Where they announce the Citizen of the Year?"

"Yes?"

"There's going to be a big surprise! They just decided the winner! You just *got* to be there. You won't believe it!"

I reeled in disbelief. *Someone else was being given the Citizen of the Year Award!*

"Who's getting the award?"

"I'm not supposed to tell you."

"Tell me!"

"Okay, I'll tell you but you got to act surprised tonight," he continued. "Six o'clock sharp! Bring Maya and the girls. You got to give a *knockout* speech praising Karl. *Karl's getting the award!* Isn't that great?"

I went home at four in the afternoon. To my surprise, Maya had the scoop on me.

"Karl's getting the Citizen of the Year Award! He did it!" she said.

"Actually, I knew that. He told me days ago."

"You didn't tell me!"

"There were so many other things going on."

Maya scowled, then recovered.

"And good news for you, too," she said. "Ken Patel from the motel called me and said that the investigator told him he was done and he was satisfied that there was no case against you. The investigator said he was checking out and going back to Austin."

"So our network of spies is fully functional," I said with a laugh.

"This is a small town, and everyone knows everything."

"Kind of scary."

The girls were delighted to have me home, and we had a celebration. We had missed lunch, so we had an early dinner. Maya made grilled cheese sandwiches and fresh waffles. I made hot chocolate. The smell of burnt sugar and toasting waffles was comforting. The four of us snuggled together on the sofa.

"What happen, Dad?" Anjali asked.

"Did they say you were good? Didn't do anything wrong?" Priya asked.

"Policeman gone?" Anjali asked.

"Yes, yes. Totally cleared. The investigator hasn't gone. He's looking into another matter, but it has nothing to do with me."

"Yay, Dad!" the girls said in unison.

"And, wonder of wonders, guess who came up to me and apologized?"

"Who did?" Maya asked.

"Joe, the lab chief! He always gives me a hard time, but he came and told me that the investigator came into the lab and was satisfied that he was using gloves while drawing blood samples. He was only doing it because I had ordered him to do it. Joe had refused when I asked him the first time."

"And what's this about the Citizen of the Year Award?" Maya asked.

"Well, the administrator told me that I needed to be there, to give a speech for Karl."

"They're going to give Karl the Citizen of the Year Award? That's great!"

I was envious. I had to understand, Karl had been there for years, he had looked after everyone in the ER and in the hospital and the clinic, he had been the school doctor, he had travelled for all the football games, he had been a huge advocate for the clinic; he deserved this honor. I was amused by my own pettiness.

"You remember when he took us out to Scarborough Lake and got out his jet skis and all?" Maya said.

"I member!" Anjali said.

"Remember the time he came to dinner? Remember the time he covered for you when you missed the fracture?" Maya said.

"I member," Anjali repeated.

I winced. I didn't want to remember. Maya turned to the girls.

"We've been here almost a year already!" Maya said to them. "I want to know, what do you remember about this time?"

"I member *you* made waffles, Mommy!" Anjali said.

"That's right! I made waffles that first night, when we had just reached Hotspur."

"What do you remember, Priya?"

"I'll always remember Mom made us waffles and pancakes for breakfast, and she makes the best daal and roti and chicken and rice!"

"I member!" Anjali said.

"I'll always remember Mom made us do coloring outside by the garage, and made us blow bubbles there!" Priya added.

"I member!" Anjali echoed.

"And I'll always remember that Mom shampooed my hair and Anjali's hair and put it into ponytails!" Priya continued.

"I member ponies! Ponies!" Anjali said.

"I'll always remember that Mom took us swimming and told us to watch out for the dirty bathrooms!" Priya said.

"Float, don't sit!" Anjali giggled.

"I will always remember that Mom took us to school and to games," Priya added.

I was piqued. I needed to hear something.

"What about *me?* What will you always remember about me?"

"Remember about what?" Priya asked.

"About me! What will you always remember about me, your *dad?*"

Priya looked genuinely puzzled. She was at a loss for words. As she struggled for an answer, an awful realization gripped me.

"You said you will *always remember* all those things about Mom! What will you *always remember* about me?"

Priya's face brightened.

"I will *always remember* about Dad," she said, beaming, "I will always remember about Dad, *that Dad was a doctor.*"

I stared at her serene face.

I will always remember about my Dad, all I will remember, is that my Dad was a doctor.

I have never felt so ashamed in my life.

CHAPTER SEVENTEEN

With a Little Help from My Friends

I remained in a state of shock. *I wasn't the parent I thought I was.* I had told them stories at night. I had helped with some of the rituals, but I had left too many of the responsibilities to Maya. *Maybe parenting is about quantity as well as quality of time spent.* I was conflicted: I wanted to be a successful doctor, and I wanted to be a good father too, but the bitter truth was that I worked harder to be a successful doctor. I *liked* medicine. I liked the challenges, the excitement, the advances, and the prestige. I was getting better at it—and that made me work harder at it. And wouldn't my professional success help my family, too?

My primary role is that of a provider, I reasoned, *so I need to be good at my work. Our lives are better if I'm a solid doctor.* I tried hard to convince myself: *It was the right thing to do, to spend so much time in the hospital.* Yet it stung: *I'm more doctor than father.* I needed to spend more time at home. I remembered Karl asking why I didn't go home for lunch. He had known the answer: I wanted to be available to compete.

"I think it's so nice of them to give Karl the award," Maya said. "It's a big deal for him."

"I know."

"I think they are really trying to be nice to you, too."

"They're all good people. Remember when we first heard of this job opening? Remember how we felt that there would be a lot of resentment and they wouldn't welcome a foreigner?"

"Well, it wasn't just us. Lots of our friends were worried. They thought we wouldn't be welcome here."

"I remember. Julie and John were concerned, and so were the Robinsons. They thought they wouldn't welcome a foreign doctor, especially someone who wasn't white or Christian."

"But the people have been warm and very welcoming."

"It may be that they're desperate for doctors. You do fulfill a need. They really need you here."

"That's true. We all benefit. Anyhow, that doesn't take away from the fact that they have been consistently nice to us. The Templars, for instance."

"Did you know that Agatha told Priya to think of her as her surrogate grandmother?"

"She said that?"

"Yes. Priya came to ask me what *surrogate* meant. I thought it was very sweet of her."

"I guess, in retrospect, we've been lucky to end up here."

"I respect them. They love punctuality. I don't want you to arrive late for their big event tonight. I know you had a call from the ER and you have to go there first. But the dinner will start soon, and you know you have to be there to give a good speech for Karl. Be prepared, write down a few points."

"I've done that already."

"I'll take the girls and go sit with Betty, but you must be there too and *please* show up on time. Don't worry if you can't fix everything in the ER, just get things going and come. You can always go back after the presentation. Okay?"

"Okay."

"You promise?" Maya stared at me pointedly.

"I promise. I'll do my best to be there on time. The letter said that the dinner starts at six and the announcements are going to be made at seven. I'm leaving now, and I'll take my jacket. I have at least two hours, and that should be plenty."

"What's the problem in the ER?" Maya asked.

"Someone with hip pain. She used to be a Becker patient but wants to switch to me."

I tried to sound nonchalant. Maya whipped around.

"*Don't* take his patients," she said, sharply. "You *know* how that irritates him."

"Well, she's in the ER and I'm on call. I have to see her, that's all."

"You're sounding defensive."

"I am not."

"I still think you're competing with Karl."

"I'm not."

"I think you should tell Karl you're going in to see his patient."

"We don't call each other to get permission. It's understood. And he told the ER nurses that I was an academic nerd, and didn't know how to fix joint problems."

"*Do* you know how to fix joint problems?"

"Well, I did some in medical school."

"But not in internal medicine or gastroenterology!"

"True. But I can figure it out. Just to prove that I'm not an academic nerd."

"How are you going to handle this patient? It sounds difficult. Just call Karl and ask him for his advice."

I shook my head stubbornly.

"I think you're upset that Karl called you an academic nerd."

I nodded grudgingly.

"Okay. How about this: I'll see the patient and assess her. I'll do my best. If I can't help her, I will simply tell her, this is beyond me, and I will ask Karl for help. And he's going to be at the dinner, remember?"

"What if he knows her really well, like Amanda Hastings? Do you think he won't mind even then?"

"Of course he will mind! But it's a free country. If she doesn't like him, she can change doctors."

"But if it was *your* patient going over to Karl you might be saying something different, right?"

"Maybe. But right now I have very few patients, and Karl often sees them before I do, you know, if I'm running late."

"You? When *you're* running late? You don't have enough patients! Why would you run late?"

"Well, sometimes I'm tied up on the floor, with an inpatient, or in the ER."

"Please! You can break away from them for a minute. You can explain to them that you have to see a clinic patient and then you'll be right back. You need to be efficient."

"There's a fine line between being efficient and being curt."

"Be efficient tonight. And be generous to Karl! You're his colleague. The Chamber of Commerce must have thought about it a lot, and they're honoring you too, by giving you the chance to address half the county tonight. Say something really nice about Karl."

"Of course, I will! I'm not mean."

"I know, I know. You have to treat Karl with respect."

I pushed away from the table and stood up.

"I understand. I'm going to go down to the ER to take care of this patient. I'll see you and the girls at dinner."

"Don't be late!"

I walked to the door, waved goodbye to the girls, and left.

The ER was blanketed in semi-darkness. The parking lot was deserted. Inside, there was an unnatural silence and only a single overhead lamp shone. Ben Grimes stepped forward with the chart.

"Hey, sorry Doc! Fuse blew. We're on backup!"

"What happened?"

"Don't know. Last time it was a squirrel."

"A *squirrel?*"

"They get in there and chew the wires."

"Is someone coming to fix it?"

"Yep! Andy's coming! Okay, Doc, this here's Donna Sue Farley. She got her hip out of place."

I turned to look at the patient. She was in her late sixties, dressed formally in a white dress, with a halo of white hair pulled back with a rhinestone clip. She had a large red face, oversized white glasses, and bulging cheeks etched with spidery veins. She sat on the edge of the gurney, her thin legs dangling down, the left one at an unnatural angle, partially covering the right knee.

She gazed at me intently.

"You're a little one, ain't you?" she said.

"Excuse me?"

"You're a little fellow, you are! Listen, Doc, I ain't got nothing against Doc Becker. My husband Jake here, he done some dirt work for him. We used to go to the same church. But, Doc, I just got to tell you, I want to change to you. Me and Doc Becker, we got crossways, an' I ain't saying I was right and I ain't saying I wasn't. All I'm saying is, the two of us, we just don't get along. So I want you to take over."

"Well, I'm on call tonight and I'm here to help. If you want to change doctors, that's up to you. What's the problem right now?"

Jake spoke up. He was an old cowboy sitting in the corner, hunched over his wife's handbag. He had a leathery face and a white handlebar moustache. He spoke hesitantly, glancing at her for approval.

"We was going to the Chamber of Commerce dinner, and Donna Sue just got her hip outta place, Doc. Needs it pulled back in place. Happens all the time, some kinder arthritis."

Donna Sue nodded.

"Tried hip replacement, but it broke loose and then they just never could get it right again."

Donna Sue exaggerated a sad face and shook her head slowly.

"Which hip is it?"

"Left, right?" he turned to Donna Sue.

She pointed.

"Right," she nodded. "It's my left."

I drew up a stool and sat next to her. I obtained her history quickly. She was sixty-three, married, lived in Hotspur, was a housewife, suffered from hypertension and migraine headaches, and had severe arthritis of her hips, knees, feet, elbows, and hands. Left hip replacement had been attempted but failed, and the prosthesis got infected and was removed. She now had a marble-sized nugget of calcified tissue at the top of her left thigh bone, in place of a golf-ball sized sphere of solid bone. This little mass was too small to stay in the hip socket and kept slipping out.

"Have you had any other surgery?"

"Just the hip surgery. Jake?"

Jake shrugged.

"You need your hip replaced," I said. "That is way beyond my ability. I need to send you to the orthopedic surgeon in Abilene or Brownwood. Who is your orthopedic specialist?"

"Used to be Doc Brock in Abilene, but he done retired."

"His partner, then?"

"No, Doc. Listen, we got no insurance. Doc Becker just pushes it back in himself. It's real easy. Takes him just a few minutes."

"I'm not planning to treat you here. I want to send you to Abilene."

There was a chorus of protest.

"No, no, Doc! Just fix me right here! I don't want to go to Abilene! Just fix me right here!"

"Doc, I hate to push you, but they ain't gonna take her on account of we got no insurance and no money. Doc Becker generally takes her and pulls the hip back in the X-ray department. Takes him five minutes, tops."

"Doc, you can end up spending an hour on the phone or fixing me in five minutes," Donna Sue said.

I examined her, confused about my choices. *If Dr. Becker could slide it back in five minutes, so could I.* I focused on the physical findings. Her arms and legs were thin but her trunk was large, and she had a large pad of fat straddling her shoulders. Her skin was paper-thin and decorated with numerous blue blotches, especially on the forearms and hands. Her pulse was rapid, probably due to pain. Her temperature and blood pressure were normal. Her heart sounds were normal, though her heart was beating faster than the average rate. Her lungs were clear. Her neurological exam was intact. Her abdominal exam revealed a surprise: There was a large linear scar under the left rib margin. I looked up at her and asked about it.

"Oh, yeah. I forgot. Had my spleen out. Forgot to tell you, been so long."

"You had your *spleen* taken out? What for? That's a big deal."

"Doc, she had some kind of problem with her blood cells, her—her platelets, yeah, her platelets. Kind of cells does the clotting, she didn't have them. So they cut her spleen out, on account of her platelets being so low."

"Did they say she had ITP?"

"Yeah, that's it! That's it, right, honey?"

"Yeah, that's right. ITP, that's it."

Ben looked up.

"What's that, Doc? What's ITP?"

"It stands for Idiopathic Thrombocytopenic Purpura."

"Never heard of it, Doc. What is it?"

"It's a rare blood disease. *Idiopathic* means the exact cause is unknown. *Thrombo-cytes* are platelets, so *thrombo-cyto-penic* means low platelets. *Purpura* are the blue bruises that develop under the skin because of bleeding because the platelets are low. Remember, platelets are the things that help the blood to clot."

"So her blood won't clot?"

"Depends upon her platelet count now. She still has purpurae—see those blue blotches on her hands and forearms? I bet her platelet count is low. Donna Sue, do you know if the steroids and surgery fixed your low platelet problem?"

"How'd you know about them steroids?"

"Your body has all the signs of long-term steroids. You have a red face, which is a little large, and a collection of fat behind your neck, above your shoulders. Your arms and legs are thin but your trunk is, well, generous. These are clues that tell us you've been on a long course of steroids. Isn't that right?"

"Shoot! You're right on the money!"

"And I think you developed a complication of steroid therapy in your bones. It's a condition called avascular necrosis of the head of the femur, because of the long-term steroid use."

"Ooh, that's one of them hundred-dollar words. Sounds kind of familiar, Doc. Jake, is that what Doc Brock said?"

"Don't know, honey. Ain't sure."

Ben interrupted.

"Doc, let me figure this out. You said avascular necrosis. *Vascular* means blood supply so *a-vascular* means lack of blood supply. *Necrosis* means tissue's dead, so you're saying the steroids cut off blood supply to the head of the thigh bone?"

"That's exactly right! Good job, Ben."

Ben grinned.

"Not just a pretty face, eh, Doc?"

I completed my exam. The abdominal examination was normal other than the operative scar under the left rib margin. Her left hip looked deformed, with a bony protuberance on the side of her buttock where the displaced head of the femur bone had slipped out of its socket and lay pinned down between muscle layers. The left leg was bent at the knee and rotated inwards, with her left knee resting on the right knee. There were large bluish-black stains of hematomas on her left buttock, from previous dislocations and replacements. The appearance and size of the hematomas was sobering.

Ben lumbered forward.

"Doc, I still got a question. Why take the spleen out if the platelets are low?"

"That's because the spleen is where platelets are destroyed by the body. So if we take out the spleen, the destruction stops. Well, it *should* stop."

"So if she's had the steroids and they failed and then she had the spleen cut out and now she still has this bleeding under her skin—the blue blotches—does that mean that the surgery failed?"

"Yes. I think she's got low platelets again. This makes it very dangerous to pull the bone out from between the muscles and slide it back into the hip socket. It could cause a lot of bleeding in the muscles and into the hip joint itself."

"Yeah, Doc Becker got to be real careful about replacing the hip, on account of it getting jammed in her butt-ocks!" Jake sang out, cheerfully. "But we ain't worried. We got *you!*"

Suddenly, I longed for Karl to reappear and take over.

"Let's check her platelet count now, stat. How long will it take?"

"Ten or fifteen minutes."

"I'm going to my office. I'll be right back. Call me if there's a problem."

I ran up to my office to consult my orthopedic text. I unlocked the main door to the clinic and paused to adapt to the darkness. I heard Karl talking loudly on the phone, and he waved as I walked past. An emergency lamp was on. He was looking down, writing and talking with great fervor. I felt a twinge of guilt. I thought about telling him about Donna Sue, then decided against it. *I can handle it,* I told myself, *I'm on call. No need to go crying to Karl and beg for his help any time there's a challenge. She doesn't want to see him anyway.* I glanced at my watch. Five thirty. The dinner would be starting soon. My speech was at six forty-five.

I reviewed the chapter quickly. I practiced the maneuver recommended to replace the displaced hip: hold the mid-thigh area and gently rotate the femur clockwise and pull forward at the same time. I remembered the surgeon doing it in London, saying, *Steady does it, steady, steady, same tension as delivering a baby, same amount of traction.* I remembered I had done this before, in London, years ago. I remembered how quickly the tiny lady there had felt relief with that maneuver. I, again, thought of asking Karl, and hesitated near his door.

He sounded angry. *I don't give a rat's ass about the dinner. I'll tell you what to do with the award!* I peeked inside, and saw that he had turned away, his back to me, as he listened intently to someone on the phone.

Strange to see Karl actually listening to someone, I thought sarcastically. *He probably doesn't care that he is going to be late for his own ovation and award.* I waited for a few seconds, then left.

It was five forty.

Nurse Smalley sailed up to me.

"Your wife called, left a reminder: Don't be late!"

"I was expecting her to call. Tell her, thanks, I'll be there as soon as I can."

Nurse Smalley looked unconvinced. She shrugged and left.

"Ben, what about the platelet count?"

"Platelets fifty thousand."

"Her platelet count is only fifty thousand," I said. "The normal is one hundred and fifty to three hundred thousand. That means she's at high risk of bleeding. This is going to be very risky."

I looked at Donna Sue. She shrugged.

"Let me send you to Brownwood or Abilene."

I looked at Jake for support.

"Doc, we just signed that form saying we are happy staying right here. You can do it. We trust you."

This was suddenly becoming very dangerous. I had to dislodge her femur, the biggest bone in the body, by twisting and pulling it through a stranglehold of powerful muscles, drag it over the rim of the hip bone and drop the head into the socket, avoiding any bleeding. With a platelet count *a third* of the normal!

Call Karl now! a voice called out, the voice of sanity and caution. *Call him now! Right now! This is too risky!*

I ignored the voice of sanity and caution. I was giddy with excitement, short on time, and flush with a little knowledge.

"Right, let's get her to the fluoroscopy room," I instructed. "We've got to have fluoro to guide us."

I pulled a stretcher into the room and brought it flush with the examining table. Ben helped me and half-whispered, "Doc, you know we ain't got fluoro!"

"*What?*" I burst out.

"Doc, we can take still X-ray pictures real fast and Joe can shoot and develop them for you, but we don't have fluoro where they take X-rays continuously like a video camera. We got a regular X-ray camera but not the X-ray video."

"Then what does Dr. Becker do?"

"He just puts them on the table and makes adjustments and keeps getting X-rays and making more adjustments. Joe's real quick. Works fine."

"You mean I can't take X-rays while I'm adjusting something and see the picture in real time, while I'm actually doing it?"

"Doc, that's right. We don't have fluoro, just X-rays. Mind you, Joe gets them real fast."

I gritted my teeth and helped Donna Sue onto the gurney, hiding my frustration. She cried out in pain and slapped my forearm. I recoiled, stung.

"Careful, Doc," she cried. "That really hurts!"

I didn't know what to say. I was losing my patience rapidly. I paused, took a deep breath, mumbled *I'm sorry*, and resumed lifting her leg.

"Careful, Doc!" Jake repeated from the corner, but did not get up.

Ben helped me get Donna Sue transferred. She was still moaning.

"Hey, Doc, while you was up in your office, I went ahead and put in an eighteen-gauge butterfly in her vein."

"Great," I said, flatly.

"Figured you're gonna need it. On account of her needing morphine."

"Morphine?"

"Morphine. For the pain. Y'know, when you pull on her leg, she's gonna holler."

"How do you know?"

"I was there last time when Doc Becker did it. Boy, he sure did use a lot of morphine! But she sure was hollering!"

"Louder'n a stuck pig!" said Jake, chuckling and hobbling behind us, purse tucked under his armpit. "*Boy*, can she holler!"

Jake had not only come to terms with his wife's suffering, he was actually reveling in it. He went on, grinning.

"Nearly brought in all the nursing staff last time," Jake continued. "Thought we was fixin' to *kill* someone."

I stopped. The voice of reason and caution screamed *stop!*

"You know, maybe I'm not the right person to do this."

"Maybe *you* can give her enough morphine, Doc," Ben said. "Doc Becker didn't like to give her too much morphine, on account of might make her a dope head."

"Make *her* a dope head!" Jake said sarcastically.

"You hush now, Jake," Donna Sue said. "Just hush up!"

She turned to me, eyes glinting.

"I got faith in you, little doctor. You can do this!"

Joe was waiting for us in the X-ray room. He had spread a white sheet on the X-ray table and had a couple of pillows ready. He helped us move Donna Sue.

"Hey, Doc, I thought you was supposed to be at the Chamber dinner," Joe said.

"I know," I said. "But I'm on call, so I had to come here."

"That's mighty fine of you, Doc," Joe said, "but you know they need you there, can't do the awards ceremony without your nomination speech."

"I know."

"Can't say too much, mind you, but you're needed there so they can get on with it and get it done and go on home," Joe continued. "You got to give a little speech."

"I've got to do this first. She's in a lot of pain."

We positioned her carefully. Her left leg lay scrunched up, and she wriggled uncomfortably on the rigid board.

"Let's get the baseline X-ray."

"Doc Becker just goes right ahead and starts pulling!" Joe said.

"I understand. Thank you. Now go ahead and get the baseline X-ray. I want to see where we are, and I want to know where the head of the femur is, and how much it's rotated."

"Doc Becker just figures that out by feeling it," Joe pressed.

I felt a small wave of anger well up. I ignored it.

"Just do it, *please!*"

We stood behind the lead barrier as Joe took the baseline film. He whipped the film out from a chamber under the board and added, "Doc Becker would have just saved the time and gotten started."

I clenched and closed my eyes.

"Maybe."

"Doc, I'm *hurting!*"

"I understand. Ben will be right back, and then we'll get you some morphine."

"Doc, I'm hurting *now!* I need some morphine *now!*"

"Just wait a few minutes. It won't be long."

She groaned loudly and writhed again. Jake looked on, his face creased with worry.

261

"Doc, she's hurting real bad," Jake finally said. "She needs something! She ain't faking!"

Ben returned and agreed.

"Doc Becker always gives her morphine for this. I got some right here."

I was uncomfortable. I felt I was being pushed into giving her narcotics, and I resisted. I went to her side and tried to adjust her position to make her more comfortable. Had they refused to see Karl because she was a drug seeker, and was she faking her pain? Maybe he was strict and didn't give her a lot of morphine? I had heard of patients who were always looking for rookie doctors to give them narcotics. I looked at her. She certainly seemed to be in agony. I worked to keep my voice even.

"Okay, let's give her some morphine. Two milligrams."

"That's not going to cut it, Doc," Ben said. "Even Doc Becker gives her more than that."

"Let's just start with two milligrams, then we'll see. If she needs more, we'll give her more."

Joe burst into the room and rammed the wet films onto the viewing box. The films were actually wet with the developing solution and stuck to the viewing screen and shimmered. I scanned the films. There was the pelvic girdle, forming a bony ring; the right hip joint showed the head to be in the acetabulum, the deep, cup-like cavity in the pelvis. The left acetabulum was empty. The left femur lay obliquely, and I traced its shrunken head, rotated and deeply embedded in layers of dark muscle, in the upper and outer part of the thigh. I groaned.

"How bad's it looking, Doc?" Ben asked.

"Well, here's the acetabulum on the left side," I pointed out, distractedly. "And here's the head of the left femur. Or what's left of it. It's out of place and it's up here, underneath your front left pocket."

"Is it *real* bad, Doc?" Donna Sue asked again.

I looked at Donna Sue. She was wide-awake and looked back at me. I lied.

"Not too bad. Right, then, let's get started. Donna Sue, you feeling that morphine?"

"No, I'm still *hurting*, Doc, hurting *real bad!*"

"Donna Sue, the head of your left femur is out of its socket. It's twisted and slipped backward. So I'm going to have to rotate it first, to untwist it, then pull it gently forward and drop it back inside its socket like a golf ball into a hole."

"I know, but I'm *hurting!*"

I looked at the X-rays and saw my reflection. I saw the blazer, the blue tie from the Royal College of Physicians of England, the slicked-back hair, and the glistening face. I remembered London, and I thought of the surgeons there, who had always had fluoroscopy while performing this procedure. Here I was in rural Texas, thousands of miles away, doing my imitation of a competent surgeon. *Was I losing my sense of compassion?*

"Right. Right, then," I said. "Let's give her another four of morphine."

I took off my blazer and hung it on the view box and rolled up my sleeves. I put on a lead shield and strapped a thyroid shield around my neck. I slipped on a face shield and went to Donna Sue's side.

"Donna Sue, I'm going to hold your thigh just above the knee and turn it outward. Then I'm going to pull it gently toward me."

"Doc, is it going to hurt her?" Jake asked.

"I've just given her another four of morphine. That makes six milligrams in all, and that's a lot. That's how much we give for a heart attack."

Jake came to my side and nodded anxiously. I snapped on gloves, and, standing by her side, grasped her lower thigh with both hands. It was much heavier than I had expected. Surprised, I let it down gently. I gathered my strength and lifted her again. She screamed with pain; I set it down hastily. I had great difficulty holding and rotating her thigh. Within seconds, my back and arms were aching, and I was getting nowhere. Donna Sue cried out again and again. I pulled her thigh onto my chest for leverage and held it closely, and twisted my body. Donna Sue whooped loudly. I kept pulling and felt a little give. I struggled to maintain the traction.

"Take the film!" I gasped.

Joe rushed in and brought the X-ray projector down and adjusted it. He stepped back behind the screen and called out, "X-ray!" rushed back, pulled out the film from under the patient, and vanished. I relaxed the tension and immediately felt the femur slip back into the muscles. I slumped.

Nelda Smalley appeared at the door.

"Your wife called again."

"Tell her I'll be there soon as I can."

"How soon?"

"I don't know. I'll come soon as I can, okay?"

I was angry and frustrated. I was late to give my speech. *But what was I supposed to do?* Leave Donna Sue on the X-ray table? Rush off and eat a nice big dinner and leave her writhing while I give a speech?

"Doc, I'm hurting! I'm hurting real bad!"

"I just gave you six of morphine."

"It ain't touching it, Doc! I need more!"

"We give that much for a heart attack, Donna Sue."

"Doc, I'm hurting, hurting, *hurting!*"

"Didn't you hear a word she just said?" Jake grabbed my arm and shook it.

I looked at him and Donna Sue. They both had tears in their eyes and looked miserable. I felt a sense of exhaustion and defeat, and struggled to contain myself.

"Give her another four of morphine," I ordered. "Do we have Narcan nearby?"

"Yep, sure do," Ben replied, "but it's in the ER."

"No, get it here. It's the antidote to morphine, in case she stops breathing with the morphine. We have to have it here, drawn up and ready to give!"

"We got just a couple amps of Narcan. Rest is expired. If we draw it up and don't end up using it, then we got to throw it away and we won't have any more left in the hospital."

"Okay, just have it in the room," I said. "Don't draw it up, just have it in the room."

I hung my head. I was very late for the Chamber dinner, and I imagined Maya and the girls sitting there, waiting for me, explaining my absence to everyone, making feeble excuses that no one would believe. I thought of how remote we were, fifty miles from some more Narcan, how there was no fluoroscopy, how Donna Sue had a dislocated hip, and how I was trying with all my strength to pull it back into place, and failing.

Joe came back with the film and yanked my blazer off the view box. He peeled the baseline X-ray off the box and jammed the fresh film.

"Little bit better," he announced.

I looked at it. The head had rotated slightly and had pulled down about an inch. But I had felt it slip back right after the X-ray, so even that modest improvement had been lost. I went back to her side.

"Donna Sue, I'm going to have to do it again. I'm sorry, but it's going to hurt a lot. I'm going to give you a little more morphine and then I'll try again."

"Thank you, Doc," she said. "I know you are doing your best. Sorry you're not with your family at the Chamber dinner."

"That's okay. Let's try this again. Four more of morphine, Ben."

"You got it!"

I waited a couple of minutes for the morphine to kick in, then stepped forward again. I wrenched the limb up with both hands and brought it up unashamedly to my chest. I heaved mightily and rotated myself and then gradually pulled and twisted. Donna Sue kept squirming and slipping. The leg was heavy and awkward and kept sliding back. I ignored my back and limbs and persisted. Soon I started sweating, and it trickled into my eyes. I blinked forcefully, trying to keep it out, waiting for the femur to come loose. My shirt felt damp and my collar choked me. I kept pulling and, in desperation, twisted a little harder. Donna Sue howled instantly, her scream so sudden and intense that I dropped her leg in shock. I collapsed onto a stool and wiped my face. My arms were aching and I didn't think I had any strength left. I blinked at Donna Sue and felt utterly defeated. I sat in silence and wondered my next move. The door flung open and Karl stepped in, his face crimson with anger.

"What the *hell* is going on?"

He surveyed the room and understood immediately.

"*Donna Sue!*"

He glared at her. He turned.

"*Jake!*"

Jake crumpled instantly, whimpering. Karl stared at me with cold fury.

"And you! What in Sam Hill do you think you're doing?"

"She has a displaced hip. I'm trying to fix it."

"Why the hell didn't you call me?"

"I came past your office. You were busy."

"I didn't see you. You should have walked right in."

"I—I thought I could deal with it!"

"How? By reading a damn book?"

"I've done this before."

"Where? In Houston? Your GI fellowship?" Karl said with a sneer.

"London—"

"London! London was years ago! Hell, you ain't dealt with ortho stuff since you came to the US."

I glanced at Donna Sue. She was snoring softly, her belly rising and falling, looking like a Thanksgiving turkey on a flat platter.

"You got no clue, do you?"

I didn't answer. I was seething. I was angry about missing the dinner, I was angry about abandoning my family, I was angry about not being able to replace the hip of my patient, and I was angry about being caught out by Karl. I grabbed the thigh roughly and shuddered into position. I thrust her knee into my chest and heard her stifle a gasp. I had Ben hold her by her shoulders and pulled with all my might.

Nothing happened.

I repositioned and pulled again, with more of a twist.

No better.

I straightened up then flung myself into it again. This time I raised my right foot and pushed against the side of the X-ray table. I felt a slight movement.

"Doc Becker, should we give more morphine?" Ben asked, blatantly ignoring my authority.

"Hell, don't ask me! I ain't authorizing any morphine!"

"Should *Dr. Mathur* give her more morphine?"

"Ask him. He's the great doctor from London who can fix anything."

I winced.

"Doc Mathur, should we give more morphine?"

"Two more."

Donna Sue floated between sleepiness and pain, and kept moaning and drifting off. I tried again, ignoring my own pain. I clenched, stiffened, and twisted and pulled even harder. I held my breath and felt something. There was a sudden sickening wobble to the limb and Donna Sue wailed piteously.

"I just ordered some more morphine!"

The bulge under the muscle cuff reappeared, a little closer to the hip joint.

"I think I've moved it a little closer."

Jake was back by my side.

"Don't look heck of a lot better, Doc. Reckon we ought to ask Doc Becker?"

Karl stepped forward in triumph.

"Sandy, you look terrible. Take a breather."

I stepped back and caught my reflection in the viewing box. He was right. I looked exhausted, my face was flushed and wet. My tie was throttling me and I ripped it off.

"Don't tell me that's your damn Royal College tie!"

"It is."

"You're so damn pretentious!"

I folded it up quickly and thrust it into my pocket.

"Your angle is all wrong, an' you got no extra strength to waste, Einstein!"

I took that as an insult and scowled.

"Look, you want to get this fixed? Then get *on* the damn X-ray table yourself."

"*What?*"

"You heard me! Forget your pansy-ass Royal College books and professors! This is a real live woman in real damn distress! And she's got no damn platelets, so you better not screw this up! *Get on that damn table!*"

I stared at him in astonishment. He was serious.

"Why should I? Why would that help?"

"Because, Einstein, that's the only way you can properly roll and yank her leg down. Hold her leg, not her thigh. Hold the whole limb like one long piece of wood, and it will work."

I hesitated.

"What's the matter? Scared? Need a leg up? Royal College never tell you to get on the X-ray table?"

I hesitated.

"You waiting for the Queen to call?"

I swallowed and clambered onto the X-ray table. I crouched uncomfortably. I tried to stand and bumped against the projector.

"Move that damn thing, Joe!" Karl ordered.

I sat on bended knees astride her left leg awkwardly.

"Kneel on the side, dammit! You're not humping her leg, are you?"

I flushed and moved. I lifted up and held her whole leg straight against my side.

"That's right, hold her *below* the knee, closer to the ankle! Now, rotate and pull! Pull like you're delivering a baby!"

It was remarkably easier. The femur moved immediately, and with much less effort, I was able to feel the scalloped head of the femur scrape over the thigh muscles.

"Steady! Steady!" Karl yelled.

I maintained the tension and rotated first to the left, then to the right. *As if you're delivering a baby.*

"You're almost there! Steady!"

With an audible *pop* the head of the femur returned to its rightful place. Donna Sue let out a brief yelp of pain then exhaled loudly. Jake whooped and Ben whistled. Even Joe punched the air and shouted, "Yeah!"

I was exhilarated. I could not take my eyes off Donna Sue's face, relieved and blissful. I half-turned to find Karl's face right next to mine.

"When you can't fix something, you got to change your whole approach, okay? If it ain't working, don't just pussyfoot around, doing the same thing over and over, okay?"

He grabbed my forearm.

"*No one* knows it all. So never be too proud to ask for help."

Karl gripped my forearm tighter and shook it. He thrust his face within an inch of mine and said, "*Remember* that, Einstein!"

And he was gone.

I wrote orders for the patient to be admitted for observation. Donna Sue had received a large amount of morphine, and I wanted to make sure she didn't bleed into her traumatized muscles. I ordered a final X-ray to confirm good position, and checked it before leaving. Sure enough, the head was back in the socket, the acetabulum. I checked for other fractures and damage. Nothing.

I grabbed my blazer and tore out of the ER. I drove as fast as I could to the Chamber dinner at the high school gym. There was no parking anywhere close to the entrance, so I circled around and finally parked on brush. I jumped out and stumbled over the uneven ground, and fumbled for my tie. I slowed down a little after reaching the parking lot and managed to get my tie back on. I patted down my hair and controlled my breathing. John Abbott met me at the entrance. His scarlet face relaxed and his shoulders sagged. He threw an arm around my shoulder and walked me to my table.

"Thank God you're here!"

"I'm so sorry! I was caught up in the ER!"

"That's okay. We all know. Don't worry, Maya suggested we all go ahead and eat and have the awards *after* the dinner, and we packed your dinner. We're close to the end, and you're just in time."

We slipped into the darkened gymnasium. A soft buzz of recognition went up and followed us as we threaded our way to the front table where Maya was sitting with the girls and the Abbott family. Maya wore a cream-colored dress and had her hair up. She had worn her diamond earrings and a filigreed silver bracelet. The girls wore matching red dresses with blue stars and had their hair neatly done up with barrettes. I nodded to them in greeting and sat down, trying to get my bearings. I didn't see Karl or his family. *Maybe they're on stage already.*

"Where *were* you, Daddy?" Priya asked. "We've been waiting forever. We ate already!"

"You late!" Anjali echoed, smirking.

Maya bent forward and spoke softly.

"I told them to go ahead with the dinner and that we could do the awards later, so they did. They were very nice about the whole thing. There was some confusion at the beginning and the starting was delayed, something's going on. They just began the ceremony. I packed a lot of food for you."

"Great thinking! Thanks!"

I was relieved. I looked around the hall. I could make out at least sixty tables, all fully occupied. Banners proclaimed the Hotspur Chamber of Commerce, the Rotary Club, Kiwanis Club, Optimists Unlimited, Veterans of Foreign Wars, and the Masonic Lodge Fellowship. I recognized several of my neighbors and patients and waved and mouthed greetings to them. I waved to Tommy Teegarten and friends of Sparky Cummins. The Hastings nodded and smiled and Amanda pointed to me. The Templars were there, sitting upright and smiling. The hospital governing board was seated nearby, and Emily Youngblood waved enthusiastically.

I sipped iced tea and relaxed. I felt my pulse slowing down, and I began to breathe more easily. I looked for Karl, but couldn't find him anywhere. He had always been quick to see my patients, and was always upset if one of his patients came to see me. The last case had been a challenge, but I had eventually managed to replace the head of the femur, and I was proud of myself. I asked myself if I could have done it without Karl, whether I would have just gone back upstairs to consult

Chamberlain's Current Orthopedic Practice, Seventh Edition, and figured it out eventually.

Not in a hundred years, I concluded grimly. *Karl had made it happen. I could not have done it without him. He had shown me the right
way to do it, not my textbook.* He was a good man, a good doctor, a good
friend. He was my guide. I cleared my mind and realized that everyone
had bowed their heads. I did the same and listened. Someone was recit-
ing into a microphone.

"The Lord is my Shepherd; I shall not want. He maketh me to
lie down in green pastures: he leadeth me beside the still waters. He
restoreth my soul: He leadeth me in the paths of righteousness for His
name's sake."

The speaker paused.

"Yea. Though I walk through the valley of the shadow of death, I will
fear no evil: for thou art with me. Thy rod and thy staff, they comfort
me. Thou preparest a table before me in the presence of mine enemies:
thou anointest my head with oil; my cup runneth over."

I stole a glance at Maya. She nodded. I was excited. It was *me*, the
speaker was reading *my* thoughts! *I* did not want; *I* had been restored; *I*
had been led; *I* feared no evil. Truly, *my* cup runneth over.

"Surely goodness and mercy shall follow me all the days of my life:
and I will dwell in the house of the Lord forever."

I stood up and clapped, overcome.

"What are you *doing?*" Maya whispered. "Sit down!"

John Abbott smiled indulgently.

"Not yet, Dr. Mathur. Let them finish first. Then you can get up. But
Scripture *is* kind of overwhelming."

I sat down quietly, flushed, trembling. I was determined to calm
down. A hush fell over the audience. The president of the Hotspur
Chamber of Commerce thanked the pastor and began his address. I
realized with a start that it was the district attorney, Wentworth Teegarten. He looked like a wet squirrel, his hair parted in the middle and
slicked down, bright black eyes darting, a red bolo tie on an ill-fitting
collar. He rubbed his handlebar moustache at the end of every phrase
as if to make sure it was still there. He stood a foot back from the microphone and leaned forward, rather than moving up.

"Folks, Bernie MacAnalty sends his regrets, can't be here tonight on
account of being invited to Austin to the governor's place for something

real important. So he asked me to fill in. Folks, we're all here to honor one amongst us who has distinguished himself or herself by some extraordinary contribution to the people of this here town. We have a person to honor tonight, an' we can finally proceed because *someone* has finally made it back to this august assembly."

He was staring at me. The audience laughed.

"Just kidding, Doc. We all know you were in the ER helping Donna Sue Trammell and fixing her hip. Well done, by the way. Anyhow, we want to honor someone tonight. This individual did not grow up in Hotspur. He was—yes, it's a man—he was a native of some other parts. This medical person has worked real hard in our ER and the hospital and has done a great job due to his friendly attitude and deep knowledge. I know he hasn't been here long, folks, but the quality of the work he has done, we just felt we had to honor the man. He is married and has a family, has little children, and his beautiful wife is also an asset to this community."

He looked at me again, then looked away.

"Folks, this individual has been the subject of an investigation by the Texas State Board, and that has been a true hardship for him and his practice and for his family. We recognize that doctors are subject to a great deal of scrutiny. And we respect them for it. Anyhow, as you all know, the investigation has concluded, and the Board will take no corrective action. However, that doctor has decided to voluntarily go into rehab."

A murmur went through the crowd. I was confused. I looked at John Abbott. Was there something he hadn't told me? He looked away.

"So, folks, we all know what is happening. The State Board has investigated this fine young doctor and has made some recommendations. But I urge you to maintain your trust in him for all the hard work he has put in for us and for our hospital. I urge you to pray for him every day and every night."

There was a clamor of *hear, hear.*

"Dr. Karl Becker made a mistake. Folks, we *all* make mistakes. Dr. Karl is a great doctor, we all know that. And even great people make mistakes. Karl was chosen to be this year's Citizen of the Year, but he just withdrew his name. And he *strongly* recommended Dr. Mathur for that honor. Dr. Mathur is not even a US citizen, but on the strength of Dr. Karl's recommendations, and as Karl threatened to leave the hospital if we didn't—"

A titter.

"*Not* that I'm saying he threatened us if we *didn't* select Dr. Mathur, I'm *not* saying that. We all thought about it and we agreed. So I'm pleased to announce that the City of Hotspur has chosen to honor tonight, as its Citizen of the Year, Dr. Sandy Mathur as nominated by Dr. Karl Becker!"

John looked at me and was about to say something.

"*We honor Dr. Sandy Mathur as the Citizen of the Year!*"

I was stunned. I looked open-mouthed at John, who shrugged his shoulders and grinned. I stood up, then sat down, dazed.

"You keep standing up all the time. Wait to be called!" John said.

I was thoroughly confused. I was tired and hungry. I half stood up again. I was supposed to give a speech, and *Karl* was the Citizen of the Year. They had made a mistake. I sat down again to wait for the correction. Priya and Anjali giggled.

"Dad keeps standing up and sitting down!"

Maya was looking on, as surprised as I was.

"Dr. Becker was found to be doing drugs," John Abbott whispered. "He was stealing morphine and injecting himself. The investigator who was checking you stumbled onto it when he was checking the files and pharmacy records. *Everyone* in town already knows."

I looked up again. Someone pulled me up.

"Let's hear it for the Citizen of the Year!"

The audience stood up and clapped and cheered. I stumbled forward and reached the lectern. Mr. Teegarten seized me by my hand and shook it vigorously. He then grasped my shoulder and squeezed it with great emotion. He covered the microphone and whispered in my ear,

"You know, it was *Karl* that pushed for you to come here. We was going to give the contract to the Turkish o-b-gynecologist! I sure did want babies being born in this hospital again!"

He stepped back, clapping and smiling. I stepped forward and was dazzled by the light. I didn't know what to say. I heard someone nearby mutter, *Let's hope it's a short speech.* I tried desperately to marshal my thoughts and speak coherently. I couldn't. My mind was utterly scrambled with hundreds of images and no coherent picture. Teegarten jabbed me in the ribs.

"*Say* something!"

The audience waited politely. I could think of only one thing.

"I wasn't born in Texas, but got here fast as I could!"

They loved it. There was a pause for a few seconds, while they waited to see if I would say anything else. When I didn't, they stood up and applauded. Teegarten replaced the microphone and shook my hand and clapped me on the shoulder again and held up my hand. He handed me a plaque and a certificate. John Abbott walked me back and I sat down, still numb. I couldn't believe what had just happened. *Karl had been doing drugs? He had declined the award? He had recommended that I get it instead?* My head reeled.

People came up to me and congratulated me. The hospital board, the Templars, the Hastings, the Cummins family, and many others I didn't recognize. I was overcome with confusion and gratitude. After twenty minutes of meeting people, we left the chamber. The caterers whooped and whistled and pumped the air, and everyone smiled and cheered.

———

Later that night, Maya and I sat in the back porch and looked out into the night. There were a few clouds out and the moon came in and out. We listened to the brush, the chirp of crickets, the rustling of leaves, the occasional movement of birds in the trees, and the steady hum of a step-down transformer. We swatted mosquitoes and sprayed our feet to keep off chiggers.

"Well, the girls thought it was very funny, you standing up at all the wrong times!"

"Yes, they've even got a new game going where they bounce out of bed and stand up straight and say, *Look! I'm Dr.Mathur!*"

"Children are cruel," Maya said, with a smile.

"Why did we ever think we wanted them?"

"Don't remember."

Maya sighed. I spoke up.

"I can't believe it about Karl. Doing drugs. *That's* why he was always in the hospital. *That's* why he had to suddenly get up and go in the middle of the dinner."

"I suspected it."

"You did?"

"Ever since the dinner. When he suddenly went away. When he came back, his eyes were funny, and he had a strange look. I thought there was something wrong."

"I saw that too and the thought crossed my mind, but he was so clever and sharp, I dismissed it."

We sat in silence for a few minutes. We thought back about all our times with Karl. Now it all seemed so obvious. I remembered the time I saw him after admitting Amanda Hastings. He was probably injecting himself in his office, and I had walked in on him. I remembered him trying to hide something. I thought of Donna Sue Trammell ruefully.

"Karl helped me out in the ER today. Wouldn't have fixed it if he hadn't been there. Karl helped me come here, Karl got me this award. Maybe he also called the board on me, I don't know. Maybe he set a trap for me. Still, he's a good guy, I guess. I think every man's a mosaic, and no one is just completely good or completely bad. I owe him."

Maya nodded but said nothing

"It's going to be weird, not having him in the hospital. Abbott told me he's going to be gone for six months. I really hope he kicks this and comes back," I said.

Maya stood up.

"We have to go back inside. Time to sleep. Lots to do tomorrow."

I stood up and looked at her.

"Are your feet hurting? I may need to massage your feet."

She laughed as she got up. I remembered something.

"You know what Karl always says at the end of the day?"

"No."

"Time to piss on the fire and call in the dogs."

Maya rolled her eyes and headed back inside.

Epilogue

My practice flourished, and we stayed in Hotspur six years, three more than specified in my contract. I practiced internal medicine and gastro-enterology and started gastroenterology clinics in Abilene and in two small towns in adjacent counties. I drove over six hundred miles a week. Driving home one evening in 2001, I hit a doe. I was unscathed, but the car was mangled and the doe was killed instantly. This experience jolted me. Reluctantly, I gave up the outlying clinics, resigned from Hotspur, and set up a gastroenterology clinic in Abilene. Abilene is a larger town, serving around two hundred and fifty thousand, and was big enough for me to practice as a specialist. I still see patients in my office, perform endoscopies, and take care of patients in the regional medical center.

The Hotspur Hospital has done well. The clinic and hospital have undergone renovations and upgrades. The staff received more benefits, and Christmas bonuses were reinstated. The medical establishment is robust, which is unusual for small rural communities nationwide. The original medical staff has changed. I remain in touch with the doctors there.

Professionally speaking, I have had many good days and some bad days, but never a dull day I enjoy my work immensely, in spite of all the tumult with the changes in healthcare, the government mandates, the reimbursement cuts, and the conversion to electronic records. I've been practicing in Abilene for fifteen years, and I'm part of the medical community. There are now several other Indian American doctors, and most of them have been here many years. We stay in touch with our family in India; we call daily and visit annually.

We still have strong ties to the citizens of Hotspur and count many of them as our dearest friends. We know them personally; we know their families, their children, and their grandchildren. Bonnie sold her steakhouse and retired. Esperanza returned to Hotspur and later moved to San Antonio. Cactus and his wife passed away. Colton left Lancaster Manufacturing and works for the wind farm industry. Donna Sue and Jake are in the local nursing home. We remain very close to the Templars and their children and grandchildren; to this day, we have Thanksgiving and Christmas with them.

Karl recovered fully; he showed me what a genuine and generous person he was, and was always as direct with me as he was with everyone else. I'm particularly indebted to him. DA Teegarten did the legal paperwork for me to set up my solo practice in Abilene; Amanda Hastings coached Priya during her postgraduate studies; Emily Youngblood took Priya and Anjali horseback riding every summer we were in Hotspur; Dorothy Templar, Tommy and Agatha's daughter, sang *Ava Maria* at Priya's wedding as the other Templars sat with us in the front row. The friendships we formed during those years have endured. What began as a struggle continues today as a special relationship, bonded by memories of those six years.

Maya worked as an architect in Abilene for three years but gave it up to look after the girls and run my office. She is still my office manager. Priya met her husband at Texas A&M University, without any intervention from her parents. She lives in Iowa, and is working on her PhD in child psychology. Anjali is in dental school in Dallas and met her boyfriend while interning in a local bank.

My daughters often tell me how fortunate they are to have grown up in Hotspur and Abilene. There were many challenges for them, as they were the only Indian Americans in school at the time, but they adapted and feel completely at home in West Texas. They compare themselves with their friends who grew up in big cities, and are relieved that they evaded the painful comparisons and competition between Asian children.

Medicine is an intense profession. I find it most satisfying when I combine professionalism with compassion and a genuine interest in whatever interests my patients. For those considering a career in medicine, I hope I have conveyed a sense of how exciting and rewarding it can be, and for those already in medicine, I hope I have opened their eyes to rural practice and the dignity and kindness of those citizens. For all readers, I hope I have shared my deep respect and affection for the men and women of West Texas. They inspire me, and the purpose of this book is to honor them.

CPSIA information can be obtained
at www.ICGtesting.com
Printed in the USA
LVHW022152060621
689405LV00004B/23